PRAISE FOR EI

"This is no recipe book, it is a manual for transformation! Malcolm Saunders has given us a masterpiece of elixir alchemy to nourish and energize our bodies, clear and expand our consciousness, and gladden our hearts for our spirits to soar. In my many decades as a Taoist tonic herbalist, I have been waiting for this book. Well, the wait is over, let's all start living the 'Elixir Life'."

Dr. George Lamoureux, DAOM, L.Ac., Founder Jing Herbs

"Elixir Life is filled with unique, informative, and imaginative health beverages. Malcolm Saunders, the Superfood Alchemist, has crafted a remarkable assemblage of great tasting recipes to inspire, and promote well-being in everyone."

Robert Rogers (RH) AHG Author of the Fungal Pharmacy: The Complete Guide to Medicinal Mushrooms & Lichens of North America

"I've had the honour of working with Malcolm Saunders over the course of many years, and it's always a joy to be in his kitchen. As long as I've known him he's relentlessly pursued food as medicine, always with an emphasis on making it available to his community. Whether in his home, shop, or teaching kitchen, Malcolm mixes up modern herbal super-nutrition that somehow feels like home cooking. In Elixir Life, Malcolm shares recipes that not only deeply nourish, but also teach you the foundation for a lifetime of improvisation. Start here, and your own unique, hand-crafted recipes will follow."

Daniel Vitalis, Host of the ReWild Yourself Podcast; Founder of SurThrival.com and FindASpring.com

"In-depth and delightful... Elixir Life guides you in new ways to fuel your body and imbue your inner alchemy with the best offerings from the botanical world."

Nadine Artemis, Creator of Living Libations, author of Renegade Beauty and Holistic Dental Care

"A unique book like no other, Elixir life is an essential read for anyone interested in the art and practice of elixir crafting, daily tonic herbalism and intuitive eating. Malcolm does an amazing job of guiding the reader through defining, sharing, and exploring the nourishing aspects of what an elixir truly is - while equipping them with the skills and experiential wisdom for true ongoing success in their crafting. With a dazzling array of mouth watering recipes and stunning imagery, Elixir Life will leave the reader becoming a 'Master Elixir Crafter' in no time..."

Derek Fleming M.H., Founder and Creator of New Earth Organics & Vital Essence Herbs

"In your hands you have an enchanting, delicious collection of recipes to continue (or begin) your journey into herbalism. Malcolm demonstrates deep respect for the herbs and their traditions to show that elixirs are more than just food; they are a hobby and a passion!"

Madeline MacKinnon Founder of Natural Hormone Healing

"In his book Elixir Life, Malcolm Saunders breaks down the mystery around crafting elixir drinks into an easily digestible and user friendly format. Full of mouth watering imagery, great information and delicious recipes. You are sure to drink up these pages, finding all the inspiration and support you need to take your nourishment to the next level.

If you are new to this concept, this book will likely change your perspective on food forever! If you are familiar with elixirs already, you will gain great insight and new ideas for expanding your elixir crafting experience."

Yarrow Willard Cl.H. (Herbal Jedi) Owner of Harmonic Arts

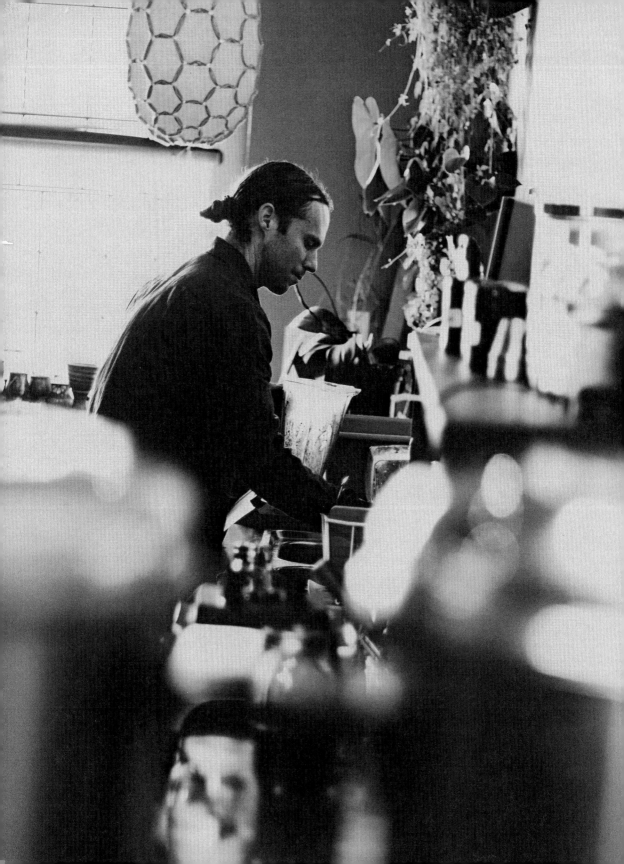

Elixir Life
Modern Nutrition Meets Ancient Herbal Wisdom

Craft Your Own Nourishing Beverages

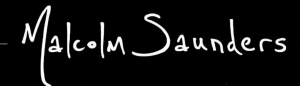

Published by Awakened Living Inc
Copyright 2018 Malcolm Saunders

ISBN (Print) 978-1-7751611-0-3
ISBN (eBook) 978-1-7751611-1-0

Editors: Marie Beswick-Arthur, Laura Milinusic & Stephaine Hrehirchuk

Photography: Jennifer Brazil, Jordan Ellams, Kendra Keir, Malcolm Saunders, Morgan Maher

Book Layout & Design by Celina Barnas

Printed in Canada.

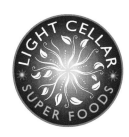

This book is dedicated to the community that is the Light Cellar.
To all staff and customers - my deepest gratitude.

FOR THE LOVE OF ELIXIRS

There is more to a delicious beverage than our tastebuds alone can sense. Beyond flavour, energy, and refreshment, it's a sacred pleasure. Elixirs provide a comforting lift, a blissful break, no matter the moment.

When you first taste an Elixir, you'll be delighted to discover something different than a typical green juice or a smoothie. An Elixir fulfills the need for energy and satisfies the desire for something deeply delicious.

They are the ultimate in everyday self-care and nourishment.

Elixirs pair the best in modern nutrition with ancient herbal wisdom. Whether the preference is to be warmed by a hot drink, or refreshed with a cool one, Elixirs answer our need for immediate nourishment and long term health.

Elixirs speak to a deeper need for us to be connected to the making of our food in such a way that it offers the opportunity for self-expression—a little creativity and inspiration to enrich our every day.

The art and craft of creating attractive, delicious, and nourishing elixirs is achievable by everyone. Along the way, crafters will feel nourished and inspired as their learning supports a delicious and easy pathway to better health.

Elixir crafting becomes a way of life as it guides, empowers, and inspires; ultimately re-creating relationships to food in a way that brings nourishing superfoods and herbal medicine into each crafter's hands and kitchen. At the heart of this process is a person's individual journey in reviving ancestral food traditions, honouring age-old cultural wisdom, while incorporating the advances in nutrition science and technology. Through this, each person can develop, re-establish, and reclaim a deeper connection with food preparation, and, as a result, strategically and intentionally nourish themselves in the modern world.

Here in ELIXIR LIFE you'll be introduced to, and become familiar with, the art and craft of Elixir making, where the best in superfood nutrition and herbal medicine is brought together.

You are about to enter a world of healing, delightful, sacred and transformative beverages...

Welcome to Elixir Life.

CRAFT THE LIFE OF YOUR DREAMS

WHAT IS AN ELIXIR?

Pronunciation: əˈliksər/

The idea of an Elixir, though ancient and mythical in origin, is finding new meaning and place in our modern world. Since its first recorded use, the definition of Elixir has varied with the popular beliefs of the time. It's interesting to see how the word 'elixir' acquired its flavour.

In searching the various meanings of Elixir, through time you might find such definitions as:

a magical or medicinal potion.

a preparation, sought by alchemists, that was supposedly able to change metals into gold.

a preparation purportedly able to prolong life indefinitely.

a homemade elixir proclaiming to enhance virility.

anything that purports to be a sovereign remedy; panacea.

an underlying principle; quintessence.

a liquid containing a medicinal drug with syrup or alcohol added to mask its unpleasant taste.

THE LIGHT CELLAR DEFINES AN ELIXIR AS:

An alchemical vehicle for the delivery of food and medicine

In this context, making an Elixir is about intentional and intelligent nourishment. You become the alchemist, bringing to life the often used, but rarely practiced, phrase of Hippocrates: Let food be thy medicine and medicine be thy food.

10 REASONS TO CRAFT AN ELIXIR

SIMPLICITY

Learning to craft Elixirs is simple. A few key ingredients added to your pantry and you are minutes away from a daily routine which leaves you feeling light and balanced; flowing easily through your day.

Between-meal-nourishment, light and uplifting: Elixirs will quickly become your favourite pick-me-up beverage for being equally delicious and simple.

SKILL BUILDING

It's super easy to make an Elixir; it's also an invitation to the exploration of a plethora of ingredients for flavours, feelings, and functional benefits. Elixir crafting opens one to the world of holistic nutrition, including a blend of herbal wisdom and current science. And its powerful... one will find an inner-sage, drawing on the wisdom of great herbal traditions and applying them for long-term benefits.

The benefits of creating and consuming Elixirs extend beyond physical health—these are ingredients which spark curiosity. Novice crafters will find themselves wanting to learn more about mushrooms, and begin to explore the less familiar with willingness. Inspiration will strike each crafter with a sense that 'this' or 'that' might be a fine balancing element to a drink—whether for flavour or function. Before long, each Elixir crafter will be experimenting and sharing with curious friends.

With a few recipes under your belt, it's a natural progression to craft your own recipes—tweaking here and there—made just for you, by you.

Elixir crafting—the art of creating healing food using the wisdom of the Earth—offers access to the path of self-knowledge.

CUSTOMIZED BY YOU, FOR YOU

Elixir Life contains all the tools, teachings, and resources needed to begin exploring new foods and herbs. Dive deep into the science, the cultural traditions, and learn from others, what foods are good for you.

Elixirs can uniquely fulfill your nourishment needs. They can play the role of aperitif, digestif, or the very meal itself. Elixirs are your morning coffee upgraded, your afternoon tea elevated, and that grab-and-go smoothie (or nutritious shake) supercharged.

When an Elixir is truly well made, it will enhance your state and nourish you on a deep level. In addition to tasting delicious, it will provide essential nutrients and energy in an easy to absorb and balanced manner.

Customizable to your mood and energy levels, Elixirs are super supportive for whatever you need and want, meeting you where you are at. Initially, you'll be choosing by name, idea, or concept. But soon you'll understand how each herb, or combination, brings a shift. Like a true alchemist, you'll choose your ingredients based on your desired experience, crafting a customized antidote for the stressors of the present moment.

An Elixir will increase your energy without the 'crash and burn' of commonly used stimulants, or it can be calming and melt away a busy day, settling the body for the night. Elixirs can also be used to help fight colds, boost immunity, and promote vibrant health.

Our younger bodies tend to be resilient and rejuvenate. As we age, we hopefully become aware of the need to nourish for tomorrow and our future years. Older bodies require diligent care. Awareness of how the small details of every day can be life-changing, and then taking action to incorporate that awareness into prevention and thriving are key to revitalization.

DEEP NUTRITION

The reasons behind the poor state of our current food system and nutritional paradigm are deep, complex, and varied.

For a long time, I have felt that something is missing from grocery store shelves. It's what eventually led me to creating the Light Cellar, a place where you can find and learn how to craft your own food and medicine.

Initially, in my teens when I began to question what I ate, I couldn't quite identify what was wrong—other than this feeling that there was something un-natural slipping into everything I consumed. Many foods were not offered as Nature intended; they missed what we truly and deeply require for living to our fullest potentials. Our current industrialized food system, though it has brought an abundance of available and relatively cheap food to our doorsteps, lacks quality, depth of character and true diversity. It also tells the tragic story of misalignment in how most of our food is grown, sourced, and prepared.

In seeking a better way of being and nourishing ourselves, we must look to the diversity offered in the wild, and by the rich traditions of the past as guides. To be deeply nourished is so much more than taking in the 'required' vitamins, minerals, and calories.

It's essential to recognize and respect the sentience and intelligence inherent in all of life, especially honouring that which we choose to consume as food.

To me, good food is also about genetics and place. The key is to incorporate a diversity of foods that exist outside the industrial paradigm, that can't be put in a box.

It's optimal, for us and for our planet, to consume foods and herbs that hold a strong life-force and genetic integrity, and which have a history of traditional use and cultural reverence.

I embrace the idea of heirloom, and choose foods that are grown on a more human scale, whether certified organic or not.

These are foods of place, from ecosystems with depth and diversity of life. They are the foods ideally tended and harvested by caring hands, with a story to tell—as opposed to fast-raised within the grips of industry.

Elixirs have been a medium through which I have found, explored, and incorporated these kinds of foods.

The unique, nourishing, and novel only add to who we are and enhance our potential in this world.

A NATURAL FOOD GUIDE

Though we certainly live in different times than our predecessors, most of the food wisdom of the past is worth preserving and reviving.

We would be wise to respect the voices and approaches of our ancestors. The past has much to teach us about the future. In the words of author and food writer Michael Pollan: "Such wisdom can right our relationship to food, perhaps more than the voices of science, industry and government." The food guides, pyramids, and groups we look to, when we wonder what we should really be eating today, are not the best resources. It's time to blend the new with old. I call this a **Natural Food Guide**. And here it is in a nutshell...

All world cultures share four distinct food/nutrient sources that can be easily brought into a simple and familiar Four Food Group format from which a helpful food-guide can be formed.

Plants ⸱⸱ Animals ⸱⸱ Fungi ⸱⸱ Bacteria

Considering these four distinct and unique food sources will naturally begin to bring more diversity into your diet and result in greater nourishment, as long as each food group is explored in depth—an endeavour easily accomplished with an Elixir.

The wide range of herbs and nutrient-rich foods which can make their way into your daily Elixir will expand your palette and open the door to new flavours and food experiences.

Culinary diversity goes beyond dietary sufficiency.

CULINARY DIVERSITY & SUPERFOODS

Superfoods are the gems of the food world, offering brilliantly simple solutions to one of modern society's hidden, but foundational, problems.

Current food systems have been developed to grow lots of food for the highest yield not necessarily the most delicious or nutrient rich. Most conventional food is too high in calories, and too low in nutrients. Tragically, food diversity today is almost non-existent, except in certain pockets of the world.

The term 'superfood' is tossed around by media and marketers. Many foods are fashionably branded as such—not unlike super-glue, super-absorbent, and super-sized.

A helpful way to approach the term 'superfoods', is to see these foods as the ones which naturally contain unique and above-ordinary properties. These properties should be validated by science, revered by culture, espoused by many, and ultimately the benefits are to be experienced by each of us.

These foods have abundant amounts of nutrients and/or unique specific nutrients. For instance, a food like Chlorella has notably high amounts of Chlorophyll, far more green than Kale, even more than Wheatgrass juice.

Superfoods are foods which blur the line between food and medicine. They are foods with a medicinal potency or herbal strength, and contain high food-value—nutrients the body needs.

To establish a perspective on this, let's look at the Apple. Leaving aside the expression, 'an Apple a day keeps the doctor away', most would not consider an Apple to be medicine, but rather a wonderfully nourishing food filled with good food value, like solid caloric value, vitamins, and minerals.

Now look at a classic example of an herb like Echinacea. This is an herb known for its medicinal strength to help boost immunity. Echinacea is extremely useful to herbalists as a medicine, but it wouldn't be considered a food. It doesn't have food value—there are very few calories in Echinacea, nor is it something one would consume often.

The Goji berry is a gem of a berry; it's considered a food and a medicine. It provides food value and nutrients, including being a complete protein, but also has an herb-like strength or medicinal action; so valued is the Goji that it's considered an herb in Chinese medicine.

What about Nettle? Would you consider it a food or herb? Of course, Nettle is a plant you can eat for its great food value, much like Spinach, but it's also an incredible food to ingest for its herbal strength, so it's both. To me it is a superfood.

We can each decide what is 'super', based on exploration and observation of which foods deeply affect our wellbeing.

The key is to build your knowledge, and personalize your research to understand the superpowers of superfoods.

EVERYDAY HERBALISM

My path—my relationship—with herbalism is individual. I apply what I learn in my own time of self-exploration and study. I don't have to learn about every herb and have all its properties memorized; that's impractical for my needs. And so I focus upon what is practical to me. May we all embrace that freedom of study.

I love the spin on the definition of Herbalism that a mentor of mine shared: that it is "the institutionalization

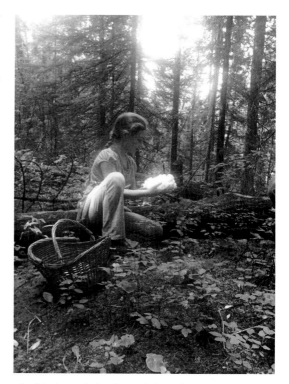

of wild plant wisdom"—a wisdom that is open to us all as we interact with elders who know and hold it, as well as through spending time with the plants themselves, both in the fields and forest as well as our own kitchen. That is how we can learn.

Herbalism has always been the people's medicine. Folk medicine, literally.

Degrees and certification have their place, but you don't need the level and formality of training of an Herbalist to practice everyday herbalism for yourself.

We are fortunate to live in a time when we have easy access to all of the herbal systems of the world. Overwhelming? Perhaps. But you can begin by choosing a few herbs that pique your curiosity.

There is a saying amongst Herbalists, with reference to their clients and prescriptions: 'the herbs don't work unless you take them'. In a more clinical manner of speaking: 'compliance is key'.

The herbs work when you take them. And, amazingly enough, they work regardless of how much you know about them. Sure, there is always the added boost of a placebo-like effect; where your knowledge and confidence in the cure brings a deeper level of healing. But you don't need encyclopedic knowledge of Dandelion to receive its benefits.

Start first exploring whatever herb(s) you are drawn to, and add to your wisdom through knowledge and experience in your own time and your own pace.

THE HERBAL ELITES - ADAPTOGENS AND TONICS

If you're starting out, why not start with the best?

Take the top five herbs of any given system, or choose a few from a number of traditions. Explore Ashwagandha and Turmeric based on what is said about them from Ayurveda. Learn about Schizandra, Reishi and Astragalus from the Chinese herbal system. Learn about Nettles and Rhodiola through the lens of Western traditions.

Whichever you choose, take them intentionally and intelligently as an essential part of practical learning—the experiential part of 'feeling and leaning' into the benefits.

It turns out that, typically, the top herbs—meaning the elite ones of any of the great herbal traditions—are not only the most powerful and effective, but also the safest to use, with the broadest range of effects on the body. These herbs are usually categorized as adaptogens and tonics. These two terms, though different, are often used interchangeably.

Donald Yance states in his book, *Adaptogens in Medical Herbalism*, that the word adaptogen refers to "the non-specific, endocrine-regulating, immune-modulating effect of certain plants that increase a person's ability to maintain optimal balance in the face of physical or emotional stress."

Adaptogens are considered helpful in counteracting any adverse effects of a physical, chemical, or biological stressor by generating nonspecific resistance.

Simply put: think of an adaptogen as something which helps one adapt to life, to stress, to any condition that arises.

Classically, tonic herbs are defined as "herbs that promote a long, healthy, vibrant, happy life, without side effects, even when taken over a long period of time." (Ron Teeguarden)

Tonic herbs have a protective, balancing, vitalizing quality beyond that of most other herbs, endowing them with the title of 'Superior Herbs' in the Chinese system.

I like to think of the concept of a tonic herb as related to the act of going to the gym to tone muscles. Just as daily exercise tones the body into better physical shape, so too does daily consumption of tonic herbs 'tonify' the body to greater health.

These two categories of herbs, adaptogens and tonics, can be used in many conditions and situations because of their beneficial effects in reducing stress.

Adaptogenic and tonic herbs differ from classically medicinal herbs. Medicinal herbs are used for a specific ailment, forcing the body or one of its systems in a distinct direction. The term dual-directional is often related to adaptogenic and tonic herbs for their ability to support the body to adapt in whichever 'direction' it needs to go. For example, there are medicinal herbs which can assist the body to raise or lower blood pressure—depending on a patient's situation. A practitioner may suggest taking, or not taking, certain herbs that have these one-directional actions. Alternatively, adaptogenic and tonic herbs can support the body to find the balance it needs—up or down, dual-directional—versus a medicinal herb taking it in one direction.

Specifically, on tonic herbs, in the words of renowned herbalist Ron Teeguarden:

"These 'Superior Herbs' are not considered to be 'medicinal' in the usual sense of the word.

They are not used to treat or even prevent specific diseases or disorders. The tonics are used to promote overall well being, to enhance the body's energy, and to regulate the bodily and psychic functioning, to protect the body and mind so as to create what the Chinese call 'radiant health.' Radiant health is defined as 'health beyond danger.' Radiant health is dependent upon one's ability to adapt appropriately and effectively to all the stresses that one encounters in the course of one's life. Tonic herbs are said to provide 'adaptive energy' which helps us handle stress much more easily."

Ron further clarifies:

"Only herbs that meet specific qualifications are ranked as tonic herbs. For an herb to be recognized as a superior (tonic) herb, that herb must have been found over many centuries of human use to meet six specific qualifications:

• A tonic (superior) herb must have anti-aging characteristics and must aid in the attainment of a long life.

• A tonic herb must have broad and profound health-promoting actions that result in a radiantly healthy life.

• A tonic herb must help balance our emotional and psychic energy so as to help improve one's state of spiritual and emotional well being and happiness.

• A tonic herb must have no negative side-effects when used reasonably, and therefore may be taken continuously over a long period of time if desired, yielding cumulative, long-term benefits. This emphasis on safety is in accordance with the first law of Chinese herbalism - 'Do no harm'.

• A tonic herb must taste good enough to be consumed easily and must be easily digestible and assimilable. Most of the herbs in the tonic category do taste good and, in fact, any of these tonic herbs may be used in healthy cooking. The tonic herbs are considered to be a major food group in the Asian diet."

Some classic examples of adaptogenic and tonic herbs are: Reishi, Ginseng, Astragalus, Goji, Schizandra, He Shou Wu, and Rhodiola. There are many others which fit this category and are to key to *Elixir Life*.

Try the herbs, learn about them, and discover how Elixirs are one of the best delivery systems for these herbs.

RECOMMENDED BOOKS:
Adaptogens: Herbs for Strength, Stamina & Stress Relief by David Winston and Steven Maimes,

The Yoga of Herbs by Dr. David Frawley & Vasant Lad,

Ancient Wisdom of Chinese Tonic Herbs by Ron Teeguarden,

Adaptogens in Medical Herbalism by Donald Yance.

THE PATH OF INTUITIVE EATING AND INTUITIVE CHEF'ING
I believe that the ultimate goal in the kitchen, beyond nourishment, is fun and freedom; total joy and liberty, mastering skills to be able to 'have, do, and make' whatever you want and need.

There is something deeply and fundamentally human about engaging one's hands in kitchen crafting and concocting. If you find your groove with it, it is as pleasurable as it is nourishing. To craft one's own food for self and others is what we as humans have done for millennia. It is natural, innate, and primal. To succeed, you need only activate your inherent wisdom and skills by continually and passionately embracing this art with your whole heart. As you do, you will feel a natural and comfortable 'knowing and flow' between yourself and your food. It is an epiphany for some to reconnect with that which has always been there: that place of inspiration and knowing-ness.

You are intuitive. You know.

Most of us have experienced what I mean by Intuitive Chef'ing— when making a smoothie, my guess is you don't need a recipe. Your intuition guides you. Elixir crafting is centered around the proficiency of Intuitive Eating and Intuitive Chef'ing.

Once a concept clicks, a recipe isn't required; the process becomes more creative and you can customize based upon ingredients on hand, and what inspires you in that moment.

When you are Intuitively Chef'ing you are creating based upon the body's needs— building a personalized recipe, not working with a recipe designed for someone else's body, pantry, and at some other place in time.

However, there is great value to starting with recipes— that's why we created this book. You can try a diversity of Elixirs, and understand how they are brought together, then, as you progress, certain ones will become your own (complete with your customization).

In *Elixir Life*, I have provided the recipe and structure, while leaving space for each individual to be led by his or her own intuition. During the process always keep in mind that which can be changed or adapted.

Don't have Reishi tea on hand? Feeling like something warming and spicy rather than cooling? Read between the lines and ingredients of each recipe and build your own.

There is a benefit—something essential and deeply human—in knowing how to prepare deeply nourishing and healing food. There is a powerful brand of caring that comes from preparing our food.

More than DIY, doing it yourself, it is what I like to call BYO—Being Your Own.

When food is literally in your hands, the connection to food becomes deeper. Appreciation grows. Food becomes sacred and connective. No longer is it something 'off the shelf' to consume.

Making chocolate from scratch will change your relationship to that food forever. This is amazing for children, because when they help make their own snack, lunch, or a treat, they gain insight, respect, understanding, and appreciation... and are much more willing to enjoy the taste.

NAVIGATING FOOD CHOICES
How unfortunate: our most basic need becomes so complicated.

These days, navigating the world of food and nutrition, trying to make the best food choices for yourself and your family, can feel overwhelming.

There is always the latest and greatest diet, as well as foods being pronounced 'good' or 'bad'. It's easy to be lured by nutrition trends, or bogged down by the dogma of opinions as they are cast about, each broadcasting 'the way'.

When reasoning through this, there are also innumerable conflicting views and bits of information coming from science and experts, not to mention the agendas of corporations, industry and advertising—all are trying, with much success, to influence what we eat.

This might be fine if access to more information and opinions did result in greater health, but for most it does not, and it often creates a longer, more frustrating and expensive journey.

I created a system to help people easily and intelligently navigate the world of food and nutrition.

It's a simple design and process based upon my own methods for evaluating any food, herb, or diet, and assessing if it is a fit.

You can apply this to know if any food, diet or nutrition information is right for you.

Use this logical and common sense approach so you can feel empowered, rather than discouraged, by all the new and changing nutrition information out there.

I call it "**FoodSCOPE**"

FoodSCOPE represents the idea of a lens through which you can view any food, herb, or diet.

The **Food S.C.O.P.E.** lenses are:

Science ·· Culture ·· Opinion ·· Personal Experiences

When confronted with a new piece of information regarding a food or diet, simply pass it through each of these lenses.

'**S**' What does Science say? What are the known and scientifically proven benefits and properties?

'**C**' How about Culture? Has this food or way of eating been practiced and consumed by any culture in the world? What, from the great culinary traditions of the world, can you incorporate that has stood the test of time in keeping a culture healthy?

'**O**' Opinions. While often helpful as a way to fast-track our success, reach conclusions, and be introduced to to new foods and herbs, the question remains: To whose opinions are you listening? What is their level of health? Can you also benefit from what they are doing, or are your circumstances too different? Perhaps their opinion doesn't mean much.

'**P.E**' Ultimately, it comes down to personal experience. How does this food or herb make you feel? Does it work? No matter what Science, Culture, or the Opinions of others are, it must be a fit for you.

Everything in *Elixir Life* has passed through the FoodSCOPE lens. The next step is for you to explore each recipe and ingredient to find the right fit for you.

THE CRAFT OF MAKING ELIXIRS

Elixir making is simple.

You can approach crafting an Elixir using a template from which to play. This 'play' equals unlimited creativity, inspired by the **flavours, feelings, and function** the crafter is looking for.

Start with pure water and make an herbal tea following the instructions for either infusing or decocting.

Place the tea (or a portion of it), strained and warm, into a blender with a healthy fat, some superfood, and herbal powders or extracts (described later), then sweeten to taste.

Blend and serve.

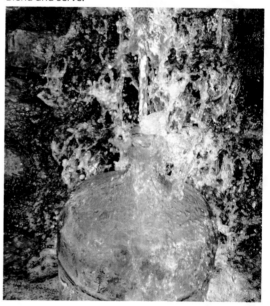

KEY INGREDIENTS

1. ALL YOUR ELIXIRS WILL BE CREATED FROM A BASE OF WATER.

It is a vital ingredient in your Elixirs to source well because this liquid becomes your blood and the delivery medium for all the nutrients. Use the best water you have access to and feel good about. We've all had the experience of drinking water that we have really liked... in fact, loved. Water so fresh, crisp and refreshing that we can't seem to get enough of it. My experience of this has been harvesting Spring water directly from the Source. I often give the analogy that drinking fresh Spring water from its source is equivalent to eating a carrot from the ground, or a tomato off the vine—no store-bought version compares. My family and I have been collecting Spring water, drinking it almost exclusively since the day we realized we could. Try it for yourself. It is transformational. This is why, for Elixirs, I suggest Spring water when available and, at the least, filtered water. To help you locate Spring water, my friend and leading health and lifestyle strategist, Daniel Vitalis, has created a website called FindaSpring.com which you can visit to find a nearby Spring for collection from the Source. There are also many high-quality water filters on the market. Look for filters that can remove chlorine and pharmaceuticals, fluoride, and heavy metals that are often found in tap water. We filter our water at home for bathing, gardening, and cooking.

2. A TEA BASE:

2. A TEA BASE: You can use any herbal tea as your base. You will see most of the recipes in this book call for Chaga or Reishi mushroom tea. At the Light Cellar they have been our staple tea bases, and we feel they offer a broad range of benefits for health and flavour as well as each being a very practical tea to brew at our bar.

For your home use choose your own teas; any you like, or are curious about. As you explore the world of herbs, discovering different flavours and benefits, you will be drawn to one or another. All good. Go with it. The base tea does play an important role in setting the tone, flavour, and direction of the drink, but not so much that you can't adjust it. So, by all means, substitute any tea you like. See 'Techniques and Terms - Getting the Most out of Your Tea' on page 16 for creating your tea, either by infusion or decoction.

3. A FAT:

3. A FAT: Adding a fat to your Elixir brings in diverse and desirable elements. First is flavour: oils and fats enrich, elevate, and extend the flavours of other ingredients, and add body to your Elixir. Fats and oils also bring deeper nourishment and energy. They are the main source of calories that make Elixirs a food. Fats also slow the absorption of the medicinal properties and nutrients in your Elixir as well as increasing absorption of any fat-soluble properties in any of your ingredients. They extend the benefits, taking it from a medicinal herbal hit to a slow, long build and ride.

We have chosen coconut butter as the fat of choice in almost all of our Elixirs. And the reasons go beyond simple practicality in the operation of our elixir bar and its dietary friendliness for most people.

The difference between coconut oil and coconut butter (also called coconut cream), is that coconut oil is only the oil, whereas coconut butter/cream contains both the oil and the fibre. If you think about coconut like almonds, is easy to understand that when you press almonds and extract the oil, you would get almond oil. It's the same with coconut oil. But you can also grind the almonds whole to get almond butter, or, in the case of dried coconut, to get coconut butter/cream.

The coconut butter contains all the goodness of the nut, including its rich, healthy fats and fibre. Each has its own use and properties. Likely you have heard coconut oil is good for cooking due to its health benefits, as well as its ability to withstand higher heat. Coconut butter, on the other hand, if used in a frying pan, will burn because of the fibre. It is best used with liquids.

Did you know that just a spoonful of coconut butter in water makes instant coconut milk? Try it. In fact, as you make the Elixirs from this recipe book, you'll see that more often than not we use coconut butter in just that way. If we want to create a creamy latte style drink we could add milk of any kind such as dairy, almond or coconut. Doing this usually lowers the overall temperature of the Elixir—that's not always wanted. So, by adding a scoop of coconut butter (or a dairy or nut butter) to your warm tea and blending it in, there is an instant creaminess that does not affect the heat of the Elixir.

This has been especially helpful for us at the Light Cellar's Elixir bar. This practicality is timesaving, and will make it easier for you at home. All of the *Elixir Life* recipes can be used with any type of fat. Some have coconut oil instead of coconut butter, or use dairy butter or ghee. You can also use coconut cream powder, which is the coconut butter in a dried, powdered form. Simply switch the butter for powder, at a 1:1 ratio. Other nourishing fats can play the above-mentioned role, but will result in a thinner, less rich and creamy consistency. Try out any of the following and see which you prefer.

Healthy Fat Choices:
Coconut oil or butter
Coconut cream powder
Dairy butter or Ghee (clarified butter)
Cacao butter
MCT oil (medium-chain triglycerides)
Nut and seed butters like Almond and Cashew butter
Olive oil
Hemp seed oil
Milk - dairy or non-dairy

4. SUPERFOOD POWDERS: from Flowers, Fruits, Seeds, Herbs, Algae, Mushrooms, Pollens and more.

This category is diverse; it's what will help distinguish one Elixir from another. There are many options for superfoods that can be added for what I call **flavour, function and feelings.**

Each Elixir has its featured ingredient(s) chosen to steer the direction of the **flavour, function and feelings**. So outstanding are these key featured foods, that you will see their bios beside the recipes throughout this book.

For instance, Mesquite powder, the nutrient-dense seed pod from the Mesquite tree, offers a nice, earthy caramel-like flavour, functionally provides lots of vitamins and minerals, and delivers a grounded feeling by working to balance blood sugar.

You will see Lucuma in many recipes. Lucuma powder is from the Lucuma fruit that has been dried and powdered. It acts as a wonderful flavour addition, providing natural, low-glycemic sweetness, functioning as an emulsifier that harmonizes all the ingredients, and providing a touch of creaminess along with a feeling of pure and simple nourishment from its spectrum of vitamins and minerals.

Some of these foods are dried in their whole form and then powdered. Other ingredients, like many of the medicinal mushrooms and herbs, have been specially prepared, extracted, and then dried and ground into a powder to make them convenient for adding to recipes while preserving their integrity and nutrition.

Herbal extracts can be made with herbs such as Astragalus, He Shou Wu, Schizandra, Mucuna, and Ashwagandha. On page 17 of this book you will read about the 'hows' and 'whys' of herbal extracts.

In the next few years, a growth of Elixir blends— pre-made and intentionally formulated mixes—will become popular. These will be superfood, herb, and mushroom powders that can be used to craft your Elixir without having to have a plethora of individual ingredients on hand.

There are benefits to both approaches: crafting with the raw ingredients or using pre-mixed blends. Pre-mixed and formulated blends allow for simplicity and ease in Elixir crafting. Choosing from a spectrum of single herbs and powders allows for increased creativity and a playful exploration of your own personalized alchemy.

Examples of some single ingredient superfood powders are Lucuma, Tocotrienols, Maca, Mesquite, Baobab, Collagen peptides, Goji berry, and Cacao powder. All are nutritious foods with their own flavour and functional benefits.

A few superfood categories that you may be less familiar with are Pollens, Medicinal Mushrooms, and Algae.

Pollens, like eggs and sperm, contain the powerful reproductive potency of Life.

As a food, many of us are familiar with Bee Pollen, which has been consumed by humans for centuries, and known to be one of the most complete and nourishing foods available. However, every flower offers a pollen with its own unique and amazing nutritional and energetic benefits.

I really love playing with pollen from Pine trees, Sacred Lotus flowers, Green tea blossoms, as well as Bee Pollen. These can be found in powder and granule form and are a very tasty, energy-enhancing and nutritious addition to anyone's diet. New Earth Organics is a company which offers a number of these plant pollens.

Medicinal Mushrooms have been utilized by humans for centuries. They are revered for their medicinal properties contained within. Today, we are able to access the potent antioxidants, immune-activating polysaccharides, and a host of other benefits contained within medicinal mushrooms, it has never been easier to integrate them into our daily life—the Elixir provides the perfect opportunity.

Medicinal Mushrooms, and their extracts, including Chaga, Reishi, Lions Mane, Turkey Tail, Cordyceps, (or multi-mushroom blends) are a great way to get a spectrum of medicinal mushrooms in one scoop. Harmonic Arts is one of the few companies supplying high-quality, dual-extracts of these medicinal mushrooms.

Algae play a role in the creation of deeply nourishing Elixirs. There are micro-algae and there are macro-algae. The macro-algae are seaweeds such as Kelp, Dulse, and Irish Moss. All of them are wild-harvested and extremely delicious. The micro-algae, on the other hand, are fresh-water, microscopic, single-celled algae. They are otherwise affectionately known as pond-scum. Containing high amounts of protein, vitamins, and minerals, micro-algae, like Spirulina and Chlorella, have been consumed by humans for many generations. Both types of algae can be added to your Elixirs.

5. EMULSIFIERS: We know water and oil do not mix. But we can force them together by using a blender, and by including foods that contain emulsifying properties. You've likely seen 'soy lecithin' listed as an ingredient in many foods—chocolate bars and ice cream. Soy lecithin is added to play the emulsifying role of harmonizing the liquids and fats, bringing and holding them together in a pleasant and palatable way. However, soy lecithin is not always the best quality of emulsifier to consume. Natural foods like Lucuma, Baobab, and Maca have emulsifying properties that fulfill this purpose, while also providing a broad range of other nourishing and delicious properties.

6. SWEETENERS: Honey, Maple, Natural Cane Sugar, Coconut Palm Sugar, Stevia, Yacon Root Syrup, Jerusalem Artichoke, Dried Fruits and their powders: Lucuma, Goji, Jujube date, Monk fruit, or Lo Han Gou. Choose your own adventure with type, quantity, and quality. We each have our preference for sweet or non-sweet. In the wise words of Mary Poppins: 'a spoonful of sugar helps the medicine go down'. It is true, many of these healing and nourishing Elixirs would not be so welcomed by the newbie, or even by a seasoned vet, without a touch of sweetness to round out the flavours.

Be open, and develop your palate. Enjoy and appreciate a wide spectrum of flavours. Don't always rely on sweet. Naturally, as we continue down our path of exploring herbs and superfoods, we will gain an appreciation for a variety and complexity of flavour.

We know that some like their coffee dark and bitter; others enjoy sweet and creamy. Such is the case with Elixir preferences. There are many earthy, woody, and other natural nuances within herbs. Embrace them. To note: bitter flavours are often stronger in medicinal foods.

When dealing with blood sugar issues, or attempting to lower glycemic intake, there are myriad strategies. Play with highlighting natural flavours and natural sweetness of foods and spices like Mesquite and Cinnamon. Include sweet tasting herbs, fruits, and berries in your tea base. This could be Licorice, Goji, or Jujube date. Their sweetness, without being sugary, will be present in your tea, reducing or eliminating the addition of sweeteners in the blending stage.

7. SALT: Its role, selection, and why it is in every recipe. Salt has been given a bad rap. With salt, it's all about quality. We are mammals and require salt—it helps maintain fluid balance, has a relationship with the transmission of nerve impulses, is critical in the

absorption of chloride, amino acids and water, and it is even involved in the role of regulating blood pressure.

It's imperative to choose and use the highest quality salt one has access to. As for quantity? It will be different for each person. Salt is essential to life and a key ingredient we should all have and use in our kitchen. It is unfortunate that salt has become misunderstood, misused, and abused by media and industry. Society has been adding too much low-quality salt to too many foods. Sure, it is added to enrich flavour but, sadly, it has been used, mainly in commercial enterprise, to entice greater consumption of certain foods.

Salt does add flavour; it brings a dish to life. It is the music for flavours to dance to. Our practice at the Light Cellar is to use only natural, unrefined, whole sea salt or rock salt. We encourage crafters to use whichever salt they enjoy and feel most connected to. Add it or do not add it. Play with the amounts—remember the palate changes over time.

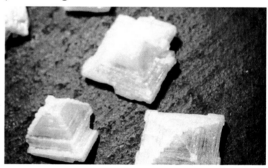

TECHNIQUES AND TERMS – GETTING THE MOST OUT OF YOUR TEA
The type of herbs with which you choose to make tea—a delicate leaf, like Nettle, or a woody mushroom, like Chaga—will determine the preparation method so as to extract medicinal and flavourful compounds with the most effective results.

INFUSIONS
Infusing is the process of steeping herbs in water to extract vital chemicals which include minerals, vitamins, sugars, mucilage, and oils. This process helps release the overall flavour profile of the selected botanical(s).

Types of herbs to use with the infusion process: Leaves, Flowers, and Berries

Examples: Green tea, Chamomile, Holy Basil, Peppermint, Raspberry leaf, Nettles...

HOT INFUSIONS

1- Place herb(s) in a pot or jar.

2- Heat water to just below boiling point.

3- Remove water from heat and pour over herb(s), cover and allow them to steep for 4-10 minutes.

COLD INFUSIONS

1- Place herb(s) in a pot or jar.

2- Fill vessel with room temperature water and allow herbs to steep 4-8 hours.

3- Strain and enjoy your cool beverage.

DECOCTIONS

Decocting is the process of simmering herbs/roots/barks in water for the desired amount of time to fully extract the properties that would otherwise not be released in an infusion.

Herbs to use with the decoction process: Roots, Mushrooms and Barks

Examples: Astragalus root, Chaga mushroom, Ginger root, Pau D'Arco bark, Rhodiola root

METHOD:

1- Pour water into a pot.

2- Add desired herbs.

3- Once the mixture comes to a boil, reduce the heat to a low simmer and cover with a lid. Allow to simmer for 20 minutes to 1 hour or longer, depending on the herb and desired strength.

4 – Strain.

Note: After straining, you may decoct the same herb(s) a second, or even a third time. You'll know no more goodness is left in the herbs as the liquid will remain clear after 're-decocting'.

STORAGE

All prepared tea can be kept refrigerated for up to a week, and reheated or used chilled.

HERB TO WATER GUIDELINES

The amount of herb(s) you choose to add to your teapot depends on the herb itself, and your intended use of the tea. These are good guidelines to work with to get you started. In our own home kitchen, I tend to grab hefty pinches for smaller, more delicate teas like Peppermint or Holy Basil that I will brew once, maybe twice. When I'm brewing bigger, more robust herbs, like Chaga and Reishi that can handle several re-brewings I'll shake the herbs in straight from the jar.

Everyday Preventative: 1-2 Tablespoons of herb to 1 litre water

Medicinal Use: 3-6 Tablespoons tea to 1 litre water

EXTRACTS:

Medicinal mushrooms and herbs can also be purchased and used in an extract form. As an extract, all the goodness from the plant or mushroom is available easily and instantly. You can add the extract, in its powdered or tincture form, directly to your Elixir, smoothie, or other recipe—its benefits can then be easily digested and absorbed.

Extracts can be made a number of ways, including through water, alcohol, vinegar, or oil extractions. We have covered how to make your own water extractions through steeping and decocting.

Alcohol extracts, known as tinctures, can easily be made at home by placing any herb at a ratio of 4:1 in a jar with 40% proof vodka and left to sit for a minimum of two weeks. This is a general method. Of course, with any herbal preparation, as you get deeper into the craft of making extracts, you can fine tune with specific ratios for each herb.

Alcohol extracts have the benefit of pulling out not only the water soluble properties of an herb, but also the non-water soluble compounds.

The method of extraction you choose will depend on the herb itself.

In fact it is often very beneficial for certain herbs to create what is called a dual-extract. This is a term you may have seen on certain products; it means that the producer has taken the herb and performed a decoction with water and an alcohol extraction. This has been done for maximum extraction of all properties, therefore potency. These dual-extracts can be found in tincture and powder form. If you are unfamiliar with the process of creating such extracts, purchasing them is the easy way to go.

You will see in many of the recipes that various herbal extracts are used for the reason of simplicity and ease. You can achieve an instant, yet potent, herbal tea by simply adding a liquid or powdered extract to water without having to go through the time and steps of its preparation. In the case of Elixirs, you can add deeper diversity of **flavour, feelings, and function** to a base drink by adding in tinctures and powdered extracts of either single ingredients, or blends.

CREATING YOUR ELIXIR EXPERIENCE: ACCLIMATIZE, SYNCHRONIZE, AND CUSTOMIZE

Acclimatize: take a moment to tune-in before you tune-up.

Ask: How do I feel?

Then create an elixir based upon those feelings.

Synchronize: look for a recipe or ingredient that resonates with your desired experience.

Customize: fine-tune your Elixir with an herbal or superfood upgrade of your choice, or choose from one of our suggestions.

You will notice that throughout the book, for many of the Elixirs, we have suggested 'upgrades'. These additional ingredients aren't essential, or part of the original recipe, but can be added for desired effect.

This concept reflects our approach to nutrition in general. That is, keep doing what you are doing, choosing the highest-quality ingredients to which you have access, and add in ingredients like superfoods and herbs that will boost your health and performance. Select them based upon desired outcome. Need to support your nervous system? Perhaps Lion's Mane... Dealing with inflammation? Turmeric with Black Pepper might be best... Need an extra lift? Cacao could do the trick...

ENHANCE YOUR ELIXIR EXPERIENCE BY CREATING YOUR OWN ELIXIR BAR AT HOME

Create your own Elixir bar at home by making the space where you will craft your Elixirs feel special and sacred. You can do this by storing your herbs in glass jars, and displaying them near your blender. In your personal Elixir bar, keep all your current favorite superfoods and health supplements, along with a few small measuring spoons—this makes adding ingredients super-efficient. Gathering your ingredients near your blender station will ensure that making Elixirs plays a part in your everyday nourishment.

TIP: Using a small basket or tray to store your ingredients and measuring spoons, on the countertop versus in the cabinet, means that you can choose to keep your current herbal favorites front of mind, and change them up as need be without over-cluttering your counter space.

A demonstration of the importance of a home Elixir bar was shared by Ron Teeguarden during one of his rare public teachings that I was lucky enough to attend at his Beverly Hills store in LA. It was a two-day training on Chinese Tonic Herbs, with far too much content to be covered in this short amount of time. Even then, Ron spent much of the first morning sharing the importance of creating a sacred space for a personal home Elixir bar.

EQUIPMENT

A high speed blender such as the Vitamix or NutriBullet RX is essential for proper mixing of ingredients.

There are various brands, designs, and models from which to choose. When I was younger, with limited income, I made do with a Magic Bullet bought online for less than a hundred dollars. These machines are affordable and efficient, and their design has come a long way. I recommend its bigger, better, successor the NutriBullet. It's an incredible high-speed blender at the right price.

Since the first time I could afford one, a Vitamix has been a key tool in my kitchen—at home and at the Light Cellar. They are much more of an investment, but their durability, warranty, and versatility are worth it. In fact, I have not found a machine that creates an Iced Alchemy as well as the Vitamix—the plunger allows the crafter to work the ingredients around the blades while blending. There are other high-speed blender models available such as Blend-tec: also good. Ultimately, it doesn't matter what you have to start with to get Elixir crafting, but at some point you're sure to want one of these upgrades.

THE LOVE OF THE MUG

Equally, part of the Elixir experience is the vessel from which you drink. To have and hold and drink from a masterfully hand-crafted piece of art is, in my mind, one of the best ways to receive your Elixir.

Of course, a glass jar or a to-go mug is sometimes the most practical. But if you are not already in love with pottery, I would highly recommend starting a collection of one of a kind mugs.

It wasn't until I married and began living with my partner, Laura, that I developed such a love and appreciation for pottery. Initially, they were gifts from friends and family, and then I started to seek out pieces. Each vessel offers its own unique character and quality, shaped by the hands and heart of its creator who crafted it through inspiration, making the world a better place through an artistic offering.

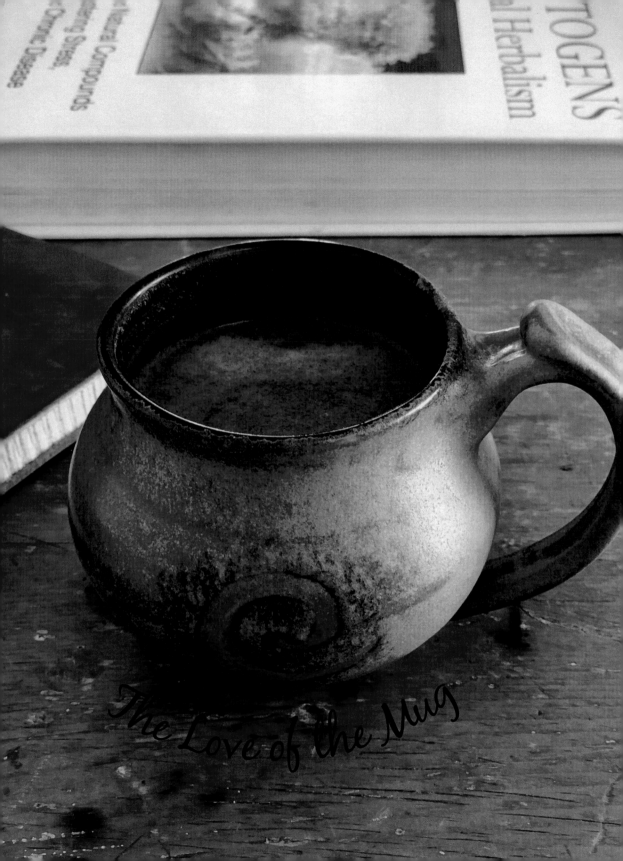

The Love of the Mug

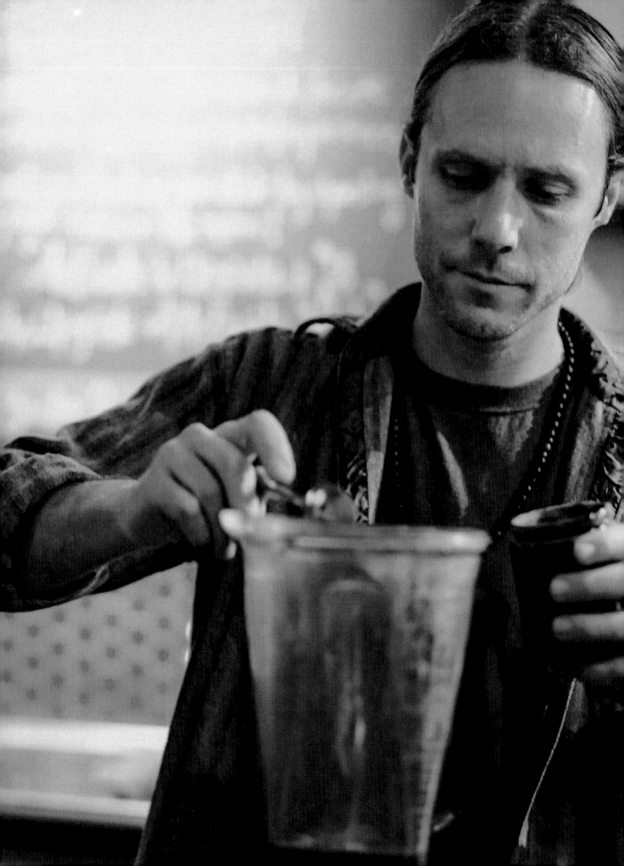

Craft Your Own Nourishing Beverages

Contributions: these recipes have been created for the Light Cellar's Elixir bar. Special thanks to our amazing staff members who have contributed in creating and upgrading each of the recipes over the years.

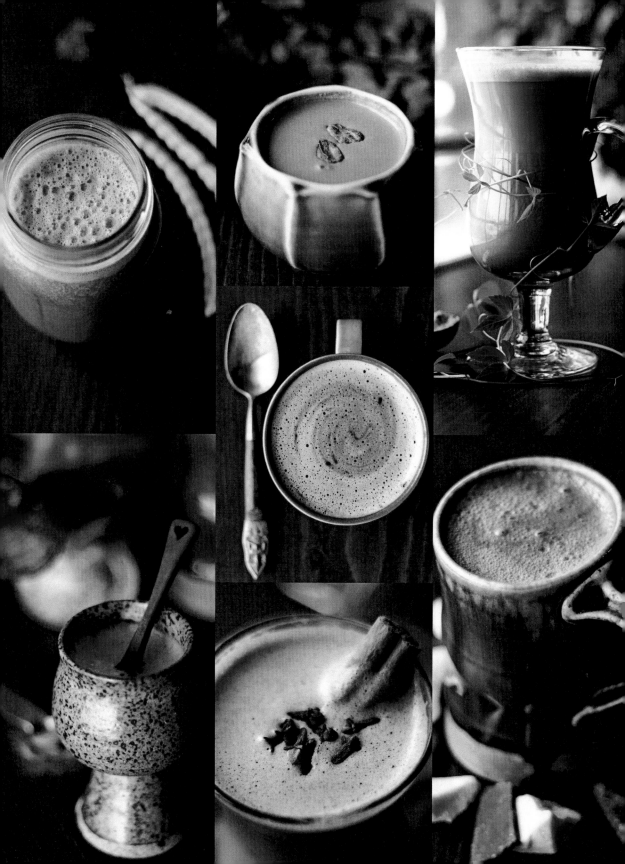

Warm Classic Elixirs

Craft Your Own Nourishing Beverages

MACA LATTE
Maca, Mesquite

ROYAL LATTE
Dandelion

CHAI SPICED LATTE
Chai Spice

LONGEVITY MACCHA LATTE
Gynostemma

CHAGA HOT CHOCOLATE
Cacao Paste

IMPRESSO
Mucuna

These elixirs are adaptations and upgrades on classic drinks you would find in a tea house or coffee shop. We took a latte and made it extraordinary. We reimagined espresso, creating a coffee-less beverage; instead, one packed with herbs that will surely impress.

MACA LATTE

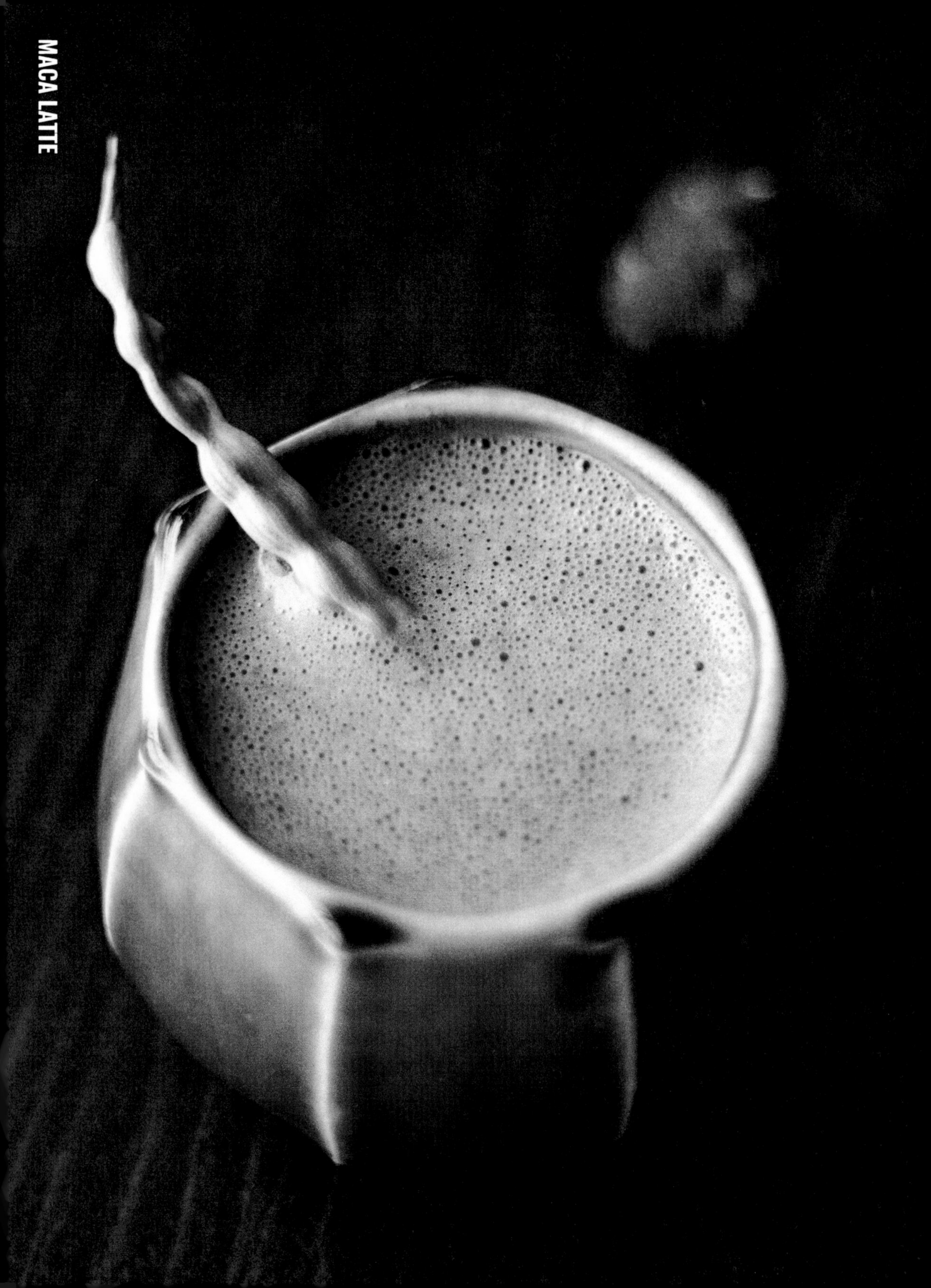

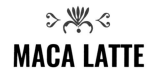

MACA LATTE

A creamy and satisfying blend of earthy flavors, crafted with Maca and Mesquite to uplift, and sustain balanced energy.

INGREDIENTS

12 ounces of steeped Chaga tea

1 Tablespoon Almond butter

1 teaspoon Coconut oil

1 Tablespoon Lucuma

1 Tablespoon Maca powder

2 teaspoons Mesquite powder

1 teaspoon Dandy Blend

1 teaspoon Maple syrup

pinch of your choice
high-quality salt

METHOD

Blend all ingredients on high with half the tea. Pour into desired cup and fill the rest of the way with hot Chaga tea.

UPGRADE

½ teaspoon He Shou Wu powder

MACA *Lepidium meyenii*

Sometimes referred to as Peruvian Ginseng, Maca is actually a cruciferous vegetable whose roots are in the radish family. This cruciferous root is high in sulforaphane, said to help the liver detoxify. Commercially, it is readily available in a dried and powdered form, though it can be found in liquid extracts and other preparations.

Maca only grows at altitudes of 2000-4000 metres. Colours range from white to black including red, yellow, purple, but, like the radish, the colour is in the skin not all the way through.

The flavour is earthy, malty, with just a hint of a radish-like spice.

Known as the 'Andes Aphrodisiac', Maca has been traditionally used to increase fertility and sex-drive as well as balance hormones. In some circles I have even heard the term, 'maca baby'- referring to those couples who used it intentionally to help create a baby.

Enjoy it in your Elixirs for its earthy flavour and a boost of energy.

MESQUITE *Prosopis spp.*

Also known as Ironwood, most people will know Mesquite from the reference to Mesquite wood-smoked or barbequed foods. However the nourishing food known as Mesquite powder is from the ground seed pod, not the bark, produced by the Mesquite tree. Traditionally consumed and relied upon as a staple food, it was revered by Indigenous peoples wherever it grew.

Mesquite is rich in fibre and protein, as well as minerals such as calcium, magnesium, potassium, zinc and iron, and the amino acid lysine.

Despite its sweetness, Mesquite is low-glycemic and has shown to be useful in helping balance blood sugars. This is due in part to its fibres, such as galactomannan gum.

Enjoy the slightly sweet, nutty, malty, caramel-like flavour of mesquite in not only this drink, but also in other Elixirs, especially chocolate-based beverages. It is one of our favourites; we are sure it will become one of yours too.

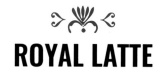

ROYAL LATTE

A coffee-inspired beverage featuring the 'King and Queen' of the Medicinal Mushrooms: Chaga and Reishi. Both of these caffeine-free mushrooms have been used as medicine for thousands of years.

INGREDIENTS

12 ounces of steeped tea ½ Chaga and ½ Reishi

1 Tablespoon Dandy Blend

1 Tablespoon Coconut butter

¼ teaspoon Reishi extract

¼ teaspoon Chaga extract

2 teaspoons Honey

2 drops Coffee Bean essential oil

pinch of your choice of high-quality salt

METHOD

Blend all ingredients on high with half the tea. Pour into desired cup and fill the rest of the way with hot Chaga and Reishi tea.

UPGRADE

Make it a Mocha.
1 teaspoon Cacao powder

Bullet-proof it.
1 Tablespoon grass-fed butter or ghee

DANDELION *Taraxacum officinale*

Traditionally used to support the healthy functioning of the liver, kidneys, spleen, and gallbladder, Dandelion is considered to be a reliable detoxifying agent, boosting the digestive and urinary systems. It is also used to calm the nerves and purify the blood, helping to lower cholesterol.

Dandy Blend is one of the easiest and most delicious ways I know of to get the benefits of Dandelion in a beverage. The main ingredient in this herbal blend is Dandelion root. Dandy Blend is a healthy and tasty coffee alternative made from the roasted roots of dandelion, chicory, and beet, as well as the extracts of barley and rye grains. It is caffeine and gluten-free, and tastes amazingly like a rich, full-bodied cup of coffee. I like to use it in recipes where I want to create a deep-rich flavour, or if I'm attempting to mimic or hint at coffee. Dandy Blend dissolves instantly into hot or cold water, offering the dark rich taste and texture of coffee, without any bitterness or acidity.

———— ◆ ————

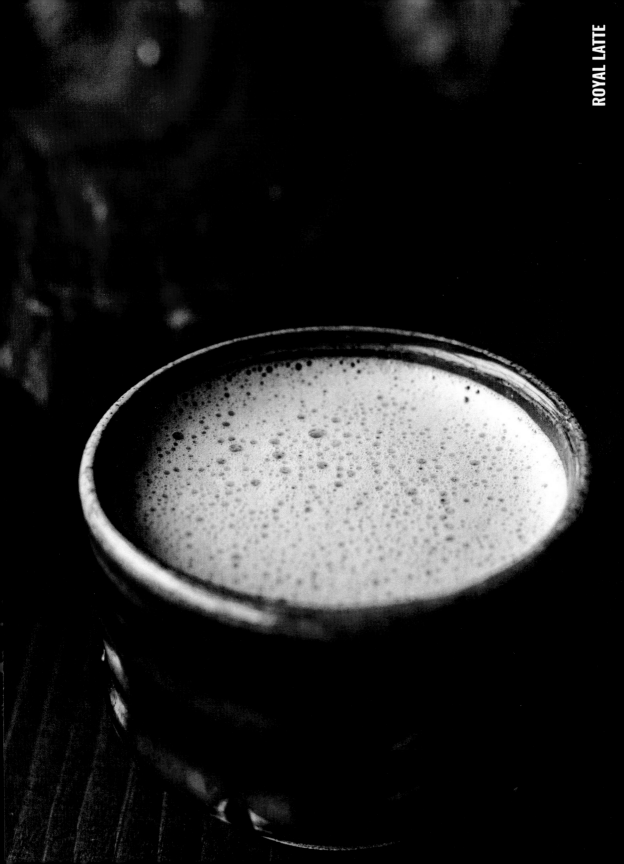

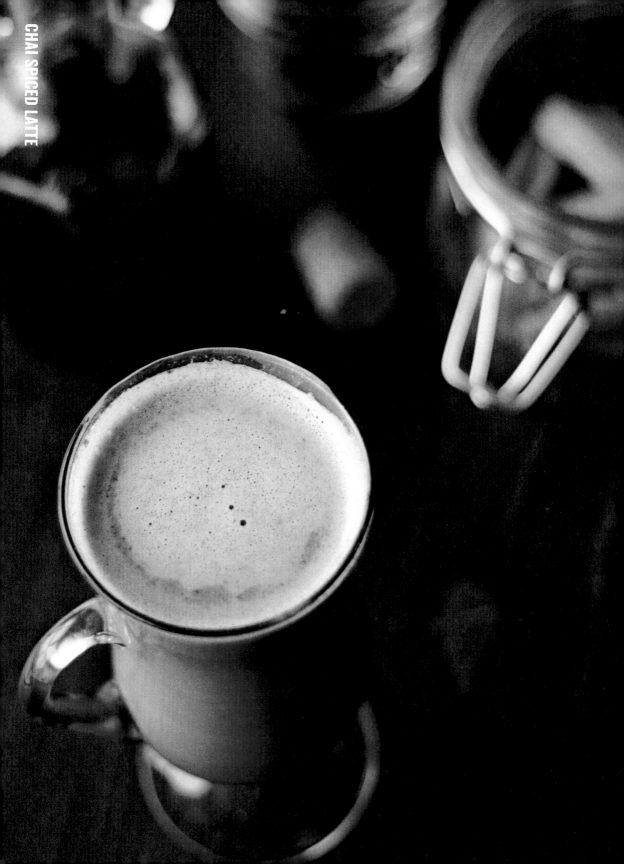

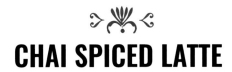

CHAI SPICED LATTE

A combination of spices to stir your inner warmth.

INGREDIENTS

12 ounces of hot Chaga tea

1½ teaspoons Harmonic Arts Chai Spice powder

1 Tablespoon Lucuma

1 Tablespoon Maple syrup

1 Tablespoon Coconut butter

1 drop Cinnamon bark essential oil

pinch of your choice high-quality salt

METHOD

Blend all ingredients on high with half the tea. Pour into desired cup and fill the rest of the way with remaining hot Chaga tea.

UPGRADE

1 teaspoon Astragalus extract

½ teaspoon Mucuna extract powder

CHAI AND THE HEALING AYURVEDIC SPICES

The feature of this Elixir is truly the healing blend of spices we know of as 'Chai spice'. Often overlooked because these spices have become so common—I think we've come to enjoy and revere the flavour more than we remember and appreciate the medicinal properties of the spices themselves.

However, in Ayurveda, and other traditions, spices like Cinnamon, Cardamom, Clove, Ginger, Allspice, Fennel, Star Anise, and Black Pepper are all known for their wonderful healing benefits.

There is also something to be said for their synergy when they come together—our universal love of Chai is testament to this.

These spices, individually and collectively, are antimicrobial, anti-inflammatory, and antioxidants, as well as aids in helping to balance blood sugar and increase insulin sensitivity.

When Laura and I travelled to India, we quickly learned that Chai means tea—as in black tea—and that Masala Chai was the name for the spiced tea that we in the West know as Chai. Similarly, Garam Masala is a common and favourite spice mix in many homes. The word garam means 'hot' or 'heating to the body', with masala again referring to a particular blend of spices. Many of the masalas or spice mixes we know and love are warming to the body, stimulate circulation, and aid digestion.

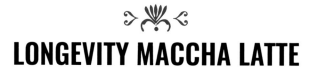

LONGEVITY MACCHA LATTE

An exquisite green tea experience that inspires one to inhale the sacredness of life.

INGREDIENTS

12 ounces of hot Gynostemma tea

1 Tablespoon Coconut butter

1 Tablespoon Lucuma

1 teaspoon Maccha powder

1 Tablespoon Honey

pinch of your choice
high-quality salt

METHOD

Place all ingredients in the blender and add in the hot Gynostemma tea. Blend until combined and serve.

UPGRADE

Ginger and Astragulus:
1 drop Ginger essential oil, ½ teaspoon Ginger powder, 1 teaspoon Astragalus powder

Minty Moringa: 1 drop Peppermint essential oil, 1 drop Spearmint essential oil, ½ teaspoon Moringa powder, ¼ teaspoon Pearl powder

GYNOSTEMMA OR JIAOGULAN *Gynostemma pentaphyllum*

Gynostemma tea is a perfect base for this Elixir because the mildly-sweet Gynostemma, which has its own flavour and benefits, allows the delicious depth of the Maccha to shine through.

Gynostemma has long been consumed daily by the peoples of the mountainous regions of Southern China and Southeast Asia. Its health-enhancing, adaptogenic and anti-aging qualities have earned its local name 'the Immortality Herb'. Those who drink Jiaogulan teas are purported to live long, healthy lives.

Known in Asia as a 'Magical Grass', this herb was said to "calm the heart and quiet the spirit." Traditionally perceived to be a cure-all, this adaptogenic herb is used to help soothe inflammation, aid digestion, and support the central nervous system. It is known to calm when one may be over excited, and it will invigorate when one is feeling low or depressed.

Also known as 'poor man's Ginseng' or 'Ginseng at tea price', Gynostemma is technically not a Ginseng, but does contain active constituents called gypenosides that are closely—structurally—related to the ginsenosides found in Ginseng, yet in a more abundant, easily accessible form.

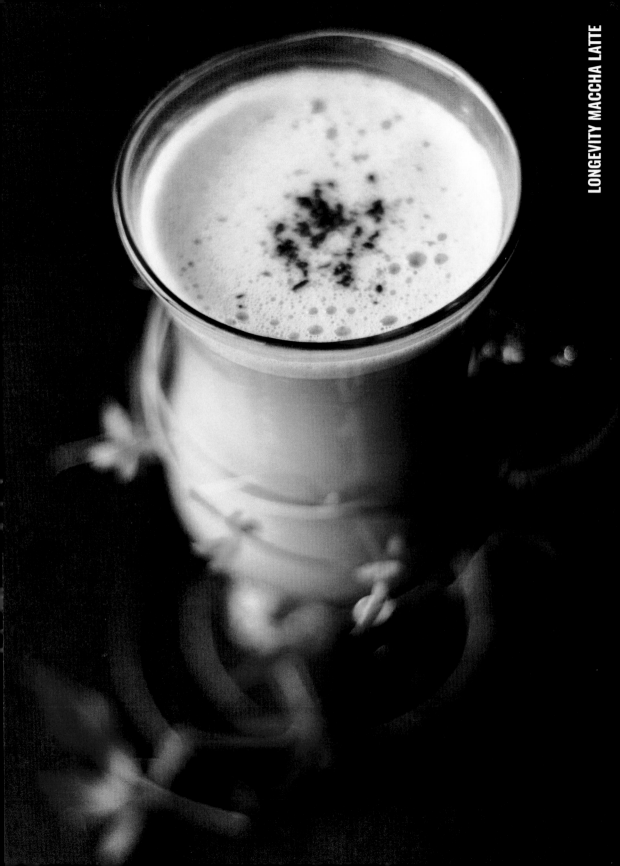

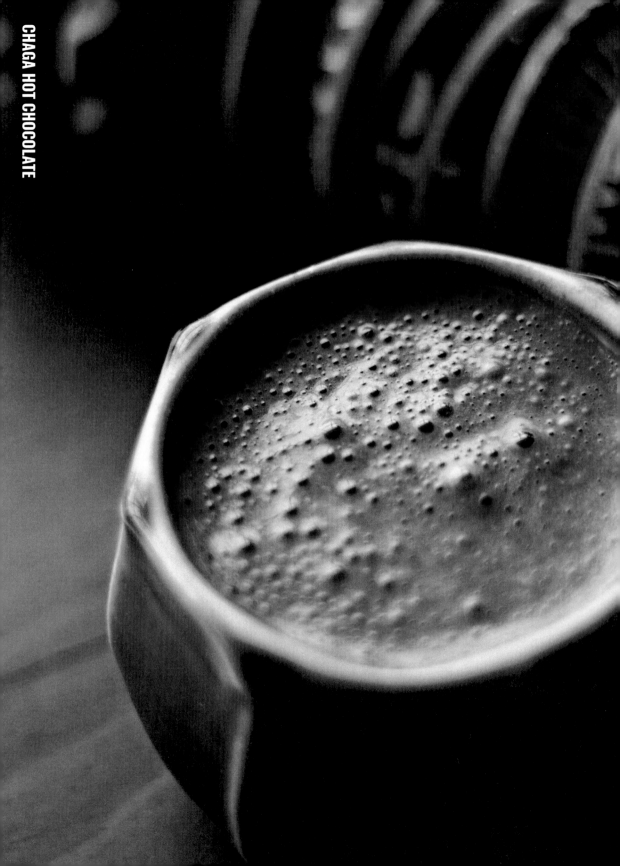

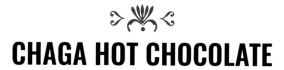

CHAGA HOT CHOCOLATE

An ultra-upgraded hot chocolate - a Light Cellar favorite in a base of Chaga tea.

INGREDIENTS

12 ounces of hot Chaga tea

2 Tablespoons Cacao paste

1 Tablespoon Cacao butter

2 teaspoons Lucuma

2 teaspoons Honey

½ teaspoon Vanilla powder

pinch of your choice
high-quality salt

METHOD

Blend ingredients on high with half the tea. Pour into desired cup and fill the rest of the way with remaining hot Chaga tea.

UPGRADE

½ teaspoon He Shou Wu powder

CACAO PASTE *Theobroma cacao*

You know when you were a kid, and you got a craving for chocolate and in searching through your parents' cupboards hunting for chocolate-anything, but all you found was the BAKERS chocolate? In those moments, I bet you thought twice about eating it. You may have asked yourself, "Do I really want chocolate?"

Essentially, what you found was Cacao paste. A dark, 100% pure chocolate, nothing else.

Also known as Cacao/or Cocoa liquor, mass, or solids, Cacao paste is the result of grinding Cacao beans into a fine, smooth paste. If you do the same with Peanuts you have Peanut butter. In the case of Cacao, you aim for an extra, extra fine and smooth consistency (like super-extra-smooth peanut butter). The reason that Cacao paste is hard at room temperature (unlike a nut that makes a nut butter) is due to its fat composition. Warmed, using a double boiler, this solid block will transform into melted chocolate—liquid gold. When Elixir crafting, Cacao paste can simply be added—in its solid form—to a hot drink, and you'll get instant rich, deep, satisfying chocolate.

VARIATIONS·

Maca: 1 teaspoon Maca powder

Mocha: 1 Tablespoon Dandy Blend, 3 drops Coffee Bean essential oil

Minty: 1 drop Peppermint essential oil, 1 drop Spearmint essential oil

Medicinal Mushroom: 1 teaspoon Medicinal Mushroom extract powder

Schizandra and Rose: ½ teaspoon freeze-dried Schizandra extract powder, 2 teaspoons Rose hydrosol

Mayan: ½ teaspoon Cinnamon, 1 drop Cinnamon bark essential oil, pinch of Cayenne

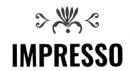

IMPRESSO

INGREDIENTS

12 ounces of hot Reishi
and Chaga tea

¼ teaspoon Reishi extract

1½ Tablespoons Colostrum

¼ teaspoon Mucuna

1 teaspoon Dandy Blend

2 teaspoon Lucuma

1½ teaspoons Coconut
Palm sugar

4 drops Coffee Bean
essential oil

pinch of your choice
high-quality salt

METHOD

Blend ingredients on high with
half the tea. Pour into desired
cup and fill the rest of the way
with hot Chaga and Reishi tea.

MUCUNA *Mucuna pruriens*

Also known as the velvet bean, and cowhage, this climbing vine grows
well in the Tropics and is native to Africa and certain parts of Asia.
Currently it is grown throughout the Tropical regions of the world to be
used primarily as a feed crop.

Mucuna has been used as an herb within many herbal traditions,
most notably Ayurveda, where it is known as Kapikacchu as well as
Atmagupta, which translates to 'secret self'. According to Ayurveda,
Kapikacchu offers many benefits—of note: it has traditionally been
used as treatment for Parkinson Disease. Today, Mucuna is regaining its
popularity and has found its way into the Elixir crafting culture.

Mucuna is best obtained as a prepared extract which has been either
hot or cold water extracted.

Used as a coffee substitute, Mucuna's flavour has been described as
'Nescafe-like'. In its extract form, simply mixed with hot water, it does
have earthy, malty, coffee-like flavour tones. It combines well with
chocolate, medicinal mushrooms, and is available to customize any
Elixirs.

As for properties and benefits: Mucuna contains high amounts of
L-dopa (levodopa), a precursor to dopamine, as well a small amount
of serotonin—all of which are involved in providing us with a happy
disposition and general sense of well-being. Many people take Mucuna
to help boost dopamine levels and experience a lift of mood through
their day.

Of course, with any herb, caution is required when pregnant or
breastfeeding. Exercise caution with this one as it has been said that
Mucuna shouldn't be used during pregnancy or while breast-feeding
because it may affect the secretion of prolactin.

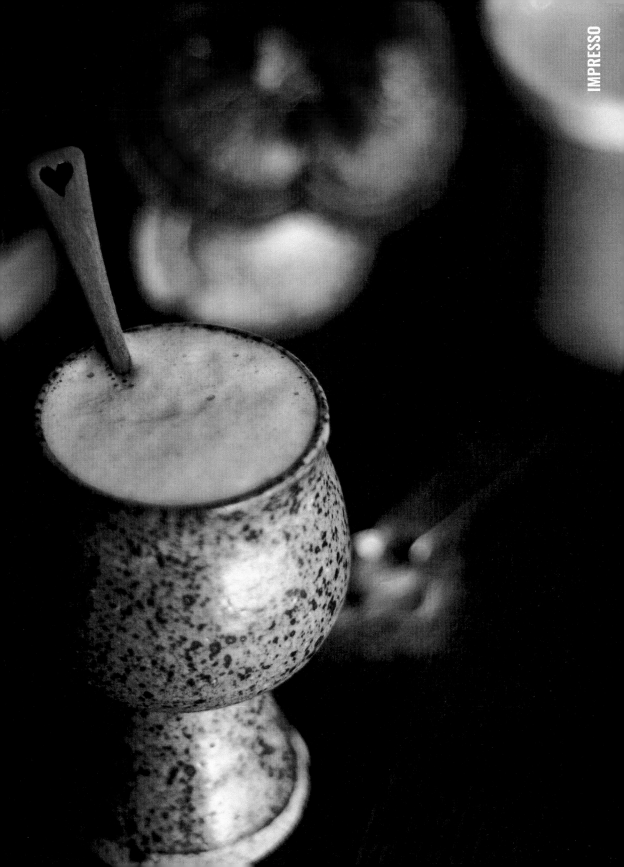

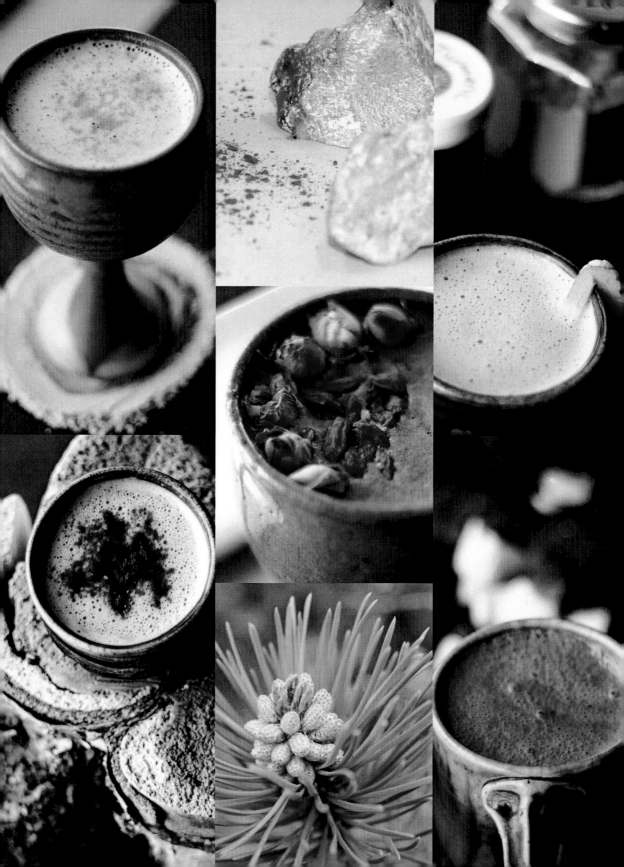

Elevated Elixirs

Craft Your Own Nourishing Beverages

TURMERIC TUNE-UP
Turmeric

HOT CHOCOLATE HEART ON
Vanilla, Cacao

BEAUTIFUL YOU
Rose

WHITE HOT CHOCOLATE MACCHA KISS
Cacao Butter

MAN ALIVE
Pine Pollen

These Elixirs are deeply inspired creations. Elevated by unique and nourishing ingredients, they fulfill a need or a wish to elevate your state—short- and long-term.

TURMERIC TUNE-UP

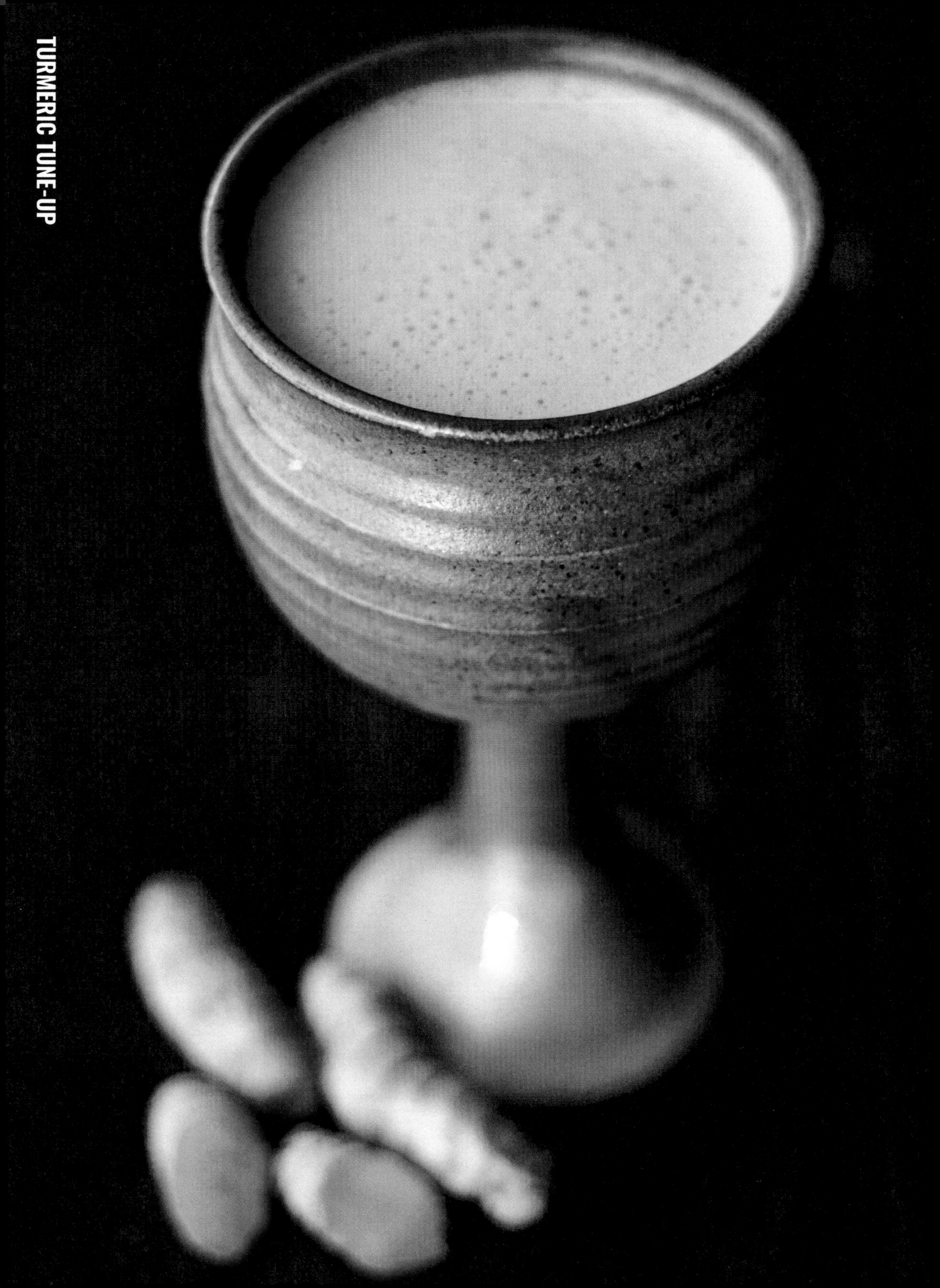

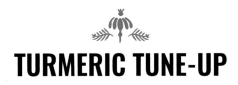

TURMERIC TUNE-UP

A botanical bounty of joy for your joints, and bliss for your being.

INGREDIENTS

8 ounces of hot Reishi tea

½ teaspoon Turmeric extract

1 Tablespoon Lucuma

1 Tablespoon Coconut butter

1 Tablespoon Honey

¼ teaspoon Ginger powder

½ teaspoon Cinnamon powder

¼ teaspoon Himalayan salt

1 drop Lemon essential oil

METHOD

Combine all ingredients into the blender along with hot Reishi tea. Blend until combined, and serve.

OPTIONAL

Top with freshly ground Black Pepper to enhance flavors and maximize the medicinal benefits of Turmeric.

TURMERIC *Curcuma longa*

Known as the 'golden spice' and 'Indian saffron', Turmeric has a very long history of medicinal use, dating back over 4000 years. In recent years it has become one of the most researched plants, with over 600 potential health benefits.

There are theories about the origin of the name Turmeric—one suggestion is that it is from the Latin terra merita which means 'meritorious earth'.

Turmeric is in the ginger family, and resembles the more familiar Ginger root. It has a distinct and vibrant yellow-orange pigment. Mirroring its ability to penetrate and stain surfaces of cutting boards and clothes, its medicinal properties are delivered deep into your tissues.

Turmeric has been touted as one of the greatest anti-inflammatory herbs due to its most celebrated active component, curcumin, which is responsible for the orange-yellow colour. The colour is also indicative of its high level of antioxidants. Among a plethora of other benefits, it helps lower cholesterol, and helps regulate and improve liver functions. There exist volumes of research and anecdotal evidence to back the claims. One point of interest, is that when Turmeric is combined with Black Pepper, it can raise blood levels of curcumin by 2000%. This is due to piperine (an alkaloid) found in Black Pepper. It's not a surprise, that, in traditional recipes, we find Black Pepper and Turmeric together—think curry and other spice blends. Piperine inhibits the body's ability to breakdown curcumin, which allows it to stay in the bloodstream longer and do its work. Another way the efficacy of Turmeric is increased when it is combined with fat, as in the case of Coconut butter in this Elixir. The Turmeric Tune Up Elixir is the perfect recipe to showcase Turmeric's qualities.

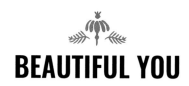

BEAUTIFUL YOU

Nourishing feminine radiance from the inside out.

INGREDIENTS

12 ounces of hot Reishi tea

1 Tablespoon Goji berries

2 Tablespoons Cacao paste

1 Tablespoon Lucuma

1 teaspoon Maca

½ teaspoon Shatavari

¼ teaspoon each of Ginger and Cinnamon powder

¼ teaspoon Pearl powder

½ teaspoon Turmeric extract

¼ teaspoon freeze-dried Schizandra extract powder

¼ teaspoon Vanilla

1 Tablespoon Honey

2 teaspoons Rose hydrosol

METHOD

Blend all ingredients on high with half the tea. Blend a little longer than usual to mince the Goji berries. Pour into desired cup and fill the rest of the way with the remaining Reishi tea.

UPGRADE

1/2 tsp Sacred Lotus Pollen

ROSE *Rosa Spp.*

Rose is said to open the heart, calm the mind, and elevate mood. All of these exquisite qualities are the reason we've added it as a key herb in the 'Beautiful You' Elixir.

The healing benefits of Rose have been known for centuries throughout many cultures around the world. For you, I'd guess, like for me, it probably only took one whiff to be wooed by its essence and transported to a place deep within ourselves.

Classically and energetically associated with the feminine, there is a quality and essence that is delicate and gentle, yet it possesses power and strength.

Among many touted health benefits, ancient cultures used Roses for digestive disorders and to ease pain from injuries and menstrual irregularities. Roses contain high amounts of Vitamin C which delivers antioxidants, supports immunity, and combats allergies. It is rich in polyphenols which are believed to be good for the heart.

Rose can be consumed as a tea from either fresh or dry petals. One of my favourite ways to enjoy this herb is as a simple Rose water—which is so easy to make and use, and captures the full-flavour and essence of Rose. Rose Water is the distilled water of Roses and is a byproduct of the production of Rose essential oil. Be sure to purchase only pure Rose water that has no added chemicals in the water, or residue from solvents used in essential oil making.

Though the use of Rose water originated in the Middle East, it has since spread around the world. Once you try it, I'm sure you'll see why.

Try adding Rose water to any Elixir in which you want to experience the uplifting qualities of this herb. Time to stop, smell, and eat the roses.

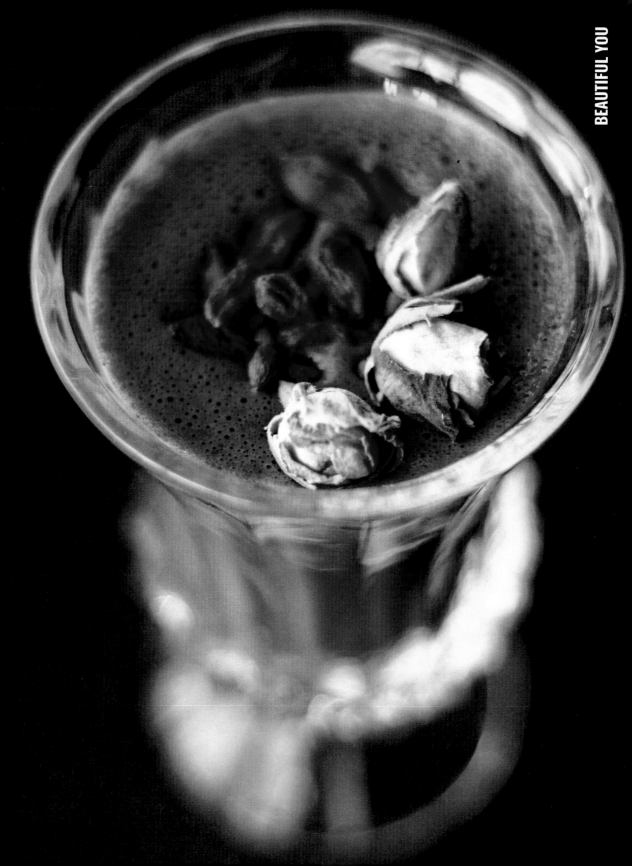

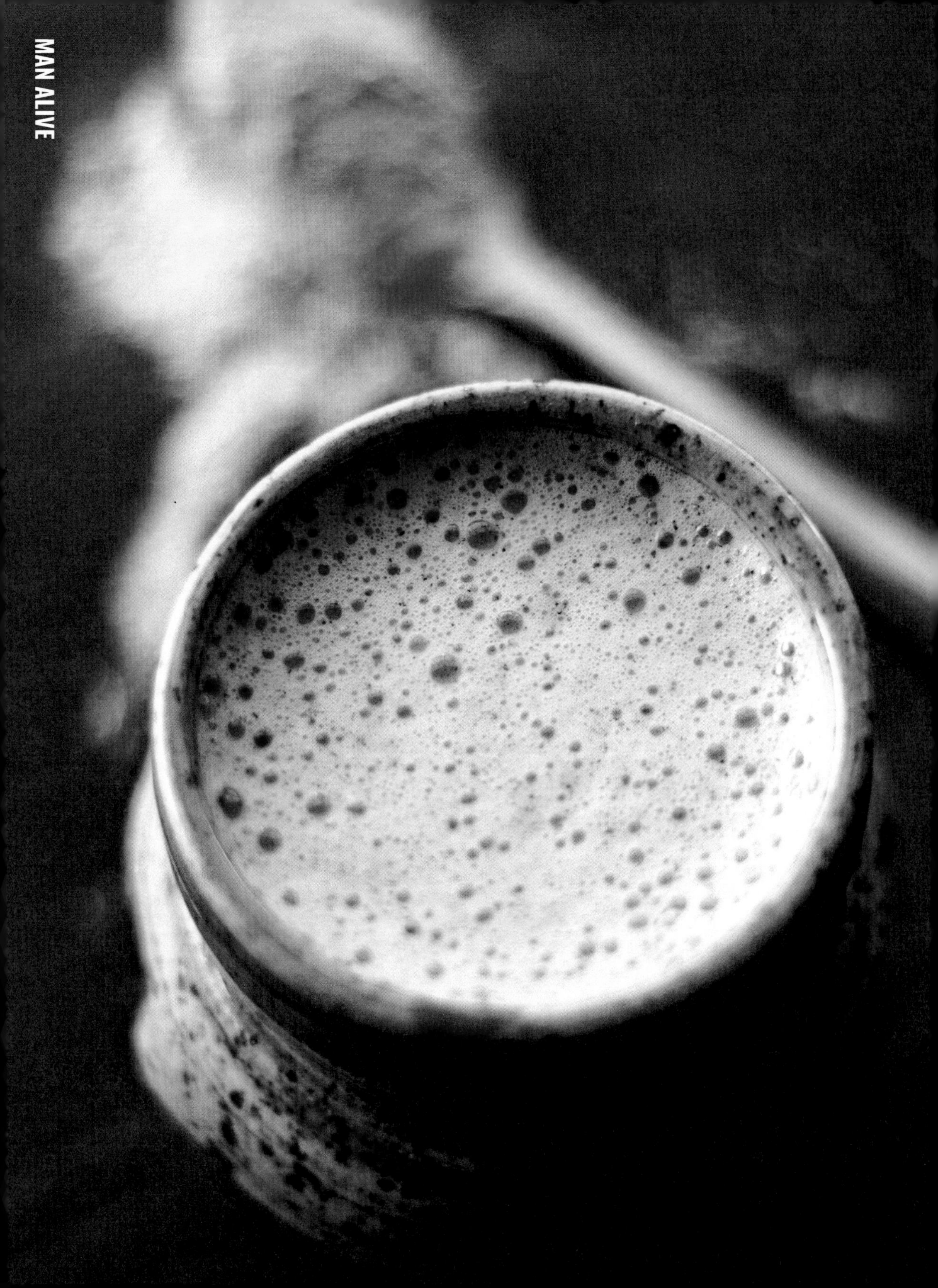

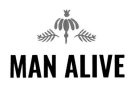

MAN ALIVE

Awaken, Energize, and Flourish

INGREDIENTS

8 ounces of hot Reishi tea

½ teaspoon Pine pollen

½ teaspoon Nettle root powder

1 Tablespoon Colostrum

¼ teaspoon Dragon Herbs TomKat

2 teaspoons Cacao nibs (optional for flavour and texture)

1 Tablespoon Coconut butter

1 Tablespoon Honey

¼ teaspoon Himalayan salt

⅛ teaspoon Cayenne pepper

METHOD

Blend all ingredients including hot Reishi tea. Pour into a mug and enjoy.

UPGRADE

1 Tablespoon Whey

1/2 teaspoon Black Mountain Ant

PINE POLLEN *Pinus spp.*

Pine pollen is a tonic, adaptogenic, nutritive, aphrodisiac, health restorative, and anti-aging superfood.

A wonderfully nutritious food, which also has well known herbal properties, the Pine pollen is from the male catkins of the Pine tree. This fine yellow powder—that seems to blanket everything around the Pine tree when it is released each Spring—provides a boost of nutrients, energy, and growth to plants and animals that come in contact with it.

Used extensively in Asia as a medicine, its earliest mention in herbal texts was by the famous Shen Nong, the legendary originator of Chinese medicine, in his *Materia Medica* (200 AD).

As a food, it comprises more than 20 amino acids, including all the essential amino acids, making it a complete protein. It also boasts an impressive array of vitamins and minerals, including B vitamins.

Pine pollen contains bio-available androstenedione, testosterone, DHEA (dehydroepiandrosterone), androsterone, and a wide variety of other natural steroidal type substances. These androgens, specifically testosterone, have been shown to increase blood levels of testosterone, and help balance the levels between testosterone and estrogen. Pine pollen's anabolic compounds have been shown to help maintain and increase muscle mass, keep the skin smooth and tight, maintain a healthy libido, optimize tissue regeneration, optimize breast health in women, support testicular and prostate health in men, aid in the excretion of excess estrogens, and speed up metabolism to help burn off excess fat.

Though I have had many male friends use Pine pollen to successfully increase testosterone levels, I know women who have also found it helpful in optimizing their health; it's not just an herb for the guys.

A fantastic book on Pine pollen is Stephen Harrod Buhner's *Pine Pollen: Ancient Medicine for a New Millennium*.

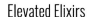

HOT CHOCOLATE HEART ON

Creamy TLC Hot Chocolate Heart On

INGREDIENTS

8 ounces of hot Reishi tea

1 Tablespoon Cacao powder

1 Tablespoon Colostrum

½ Tablespoon Cacao butter

½ Tablespoon Coconut butter

½ Tablespoon Coconut oil

2 teaspoons Honey

1½ teaspoons Rose Hydrosol

½ teaspoon Lucuma

¼ teaspoon Vanilla powder or extract

2 pinches of your choice high-quality salt

METHOD

Blend all ingredients together, then add hot Reishi tea and blend a little more.

VANILLA BEAN *Vanilla planifolia*

Known as the 'Nectar of the Gods', Vanilla is believed to have been first cultivated by the Totonacs in ancient Mexico. This member of the orchid family is a vine whose flower is, today, almost exclusively pollinated by hand. Vanilla beans are the fruit pod that is harvested and sun-cured. Though originally from Mexico, Vanilla is now grown around the world, and has several cultivars including Bourbon Madagascar, Mexican, Tahitian, and West Indian. Vanilla is the world's second most expensive spice after Saffron.

What a treat to be gifted a few pods of plump Vanilla pods; a truly decadent present and luxurious herb.

FOR THE LOVE OF CHOCOLATE *Theobroma cacao*

Chocolate is the food most associated with love.

It contains phenylethylamine (PEA), which has been dubbed the 'love molecule'. PEA is known to raise levels of endorphins (the pleasure-giving chemicals in the brain).

I came across a study, by Dr. David Lewis, which focused on brain activity when couples were kissing. He documented brain activity associated with chocolate consumption. His conclusion was, without a doubt, chocolate beats kissing, hands down, for long-lasting body and brain buzz. A buzz which, in many cases, lasted four times as long as the most passionate kiss.

Another researcher with something to say about chocolate is Dr. Terry Willard, one of Canada's leading herbalists, with over 40 years as a researcher, practitioner, and educator. I learned from Dr. Willard (and others) that we experience only a fraction of the PEA contained in chocolate; when we ingest chocolate the digestive system breaks down most of the compound, decreasing its potency and effects.

The thing is, I have a distinct memory of listening to Dr. Willard, years ago, at a conference on chocolate. He mentioned then, that research showed we have receptor sites in the roof of the mouth and that the PEA, this love molecule, can be absorbed and go directly to the brain. In this way, we receive much more of a hit from the PEA; those love feelings can feel even more sensual. Terry suggested that perhaps this explains why, the world over, chocolate lovers have a ritual of letting the chocolate melt in the mouth.

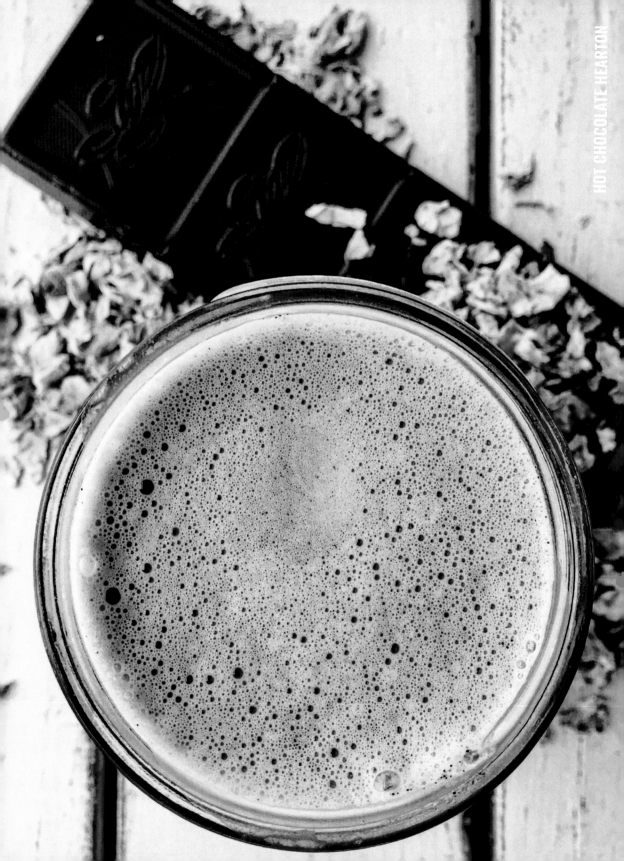

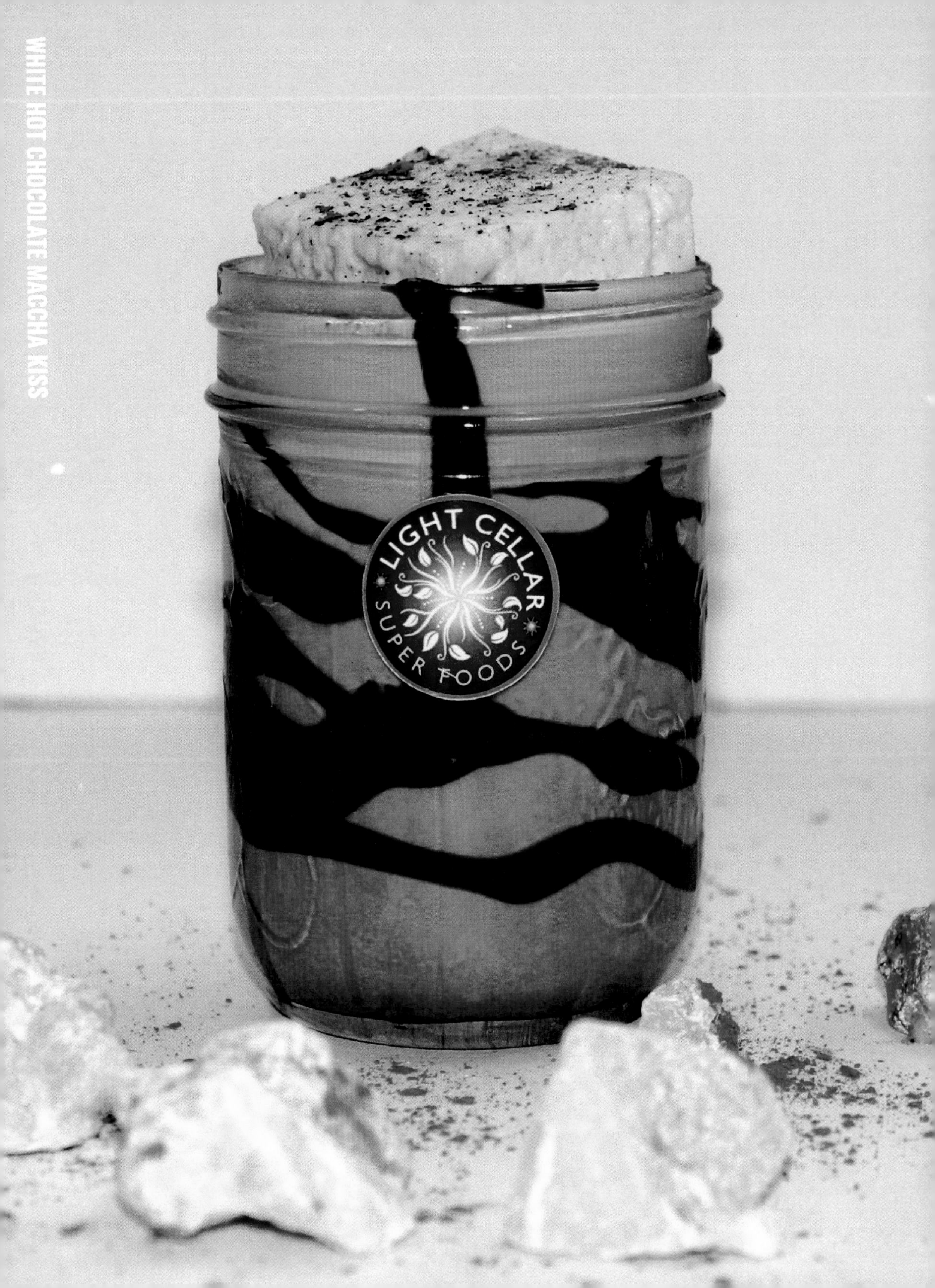

WHITE HOT CHOCOLATE MACCHA KISS

Be kissed by chocolate.

INGREDIENTS

8 ounces of hot Reishi tea

1 Tablespoon Colostrum

1 Tablespoon Cacao butter

1 teaspoon Coconut butter

1 teaspoon Coconut oil

2 teaspoons Honey

½ teaspoon Maccha powder

1 teaspoon Lucuma

pinch of your choice
high-quality salt

METHOD

Blend together ingredients, pour into a mug of choice, and top with homemade marshmallows. For further effect, pre-melt some chocolate and swirl it into your mug or glass, let chill and set against the sides. The effect creates an attractive aesthetic, as you can see in the photo, but, as the warm maccha white hot chocolate enters the glass it begins to melt the dark chocolate swirl into the beverage.

CACAO BUTTER *Theobroma cacao*

This is the fat naturally contained in the Cacao bean. It is said that a Cacao bean, depending on variety, has anywhere from 40-50% oil content. With any oil-containing fruit, nut, or seed, we can press and extract those fats—think Olive, Avocado, Hemp... It's the same with Cacao, but we call it a butter; maybe because its golden-yellow colour makes it look more like butter, but primarily because its oils are solid at room temperature. When you find and work with Cacao butter it will be in a solid state, so it requires a gentle melt in order to be worked with.

Cacao Butter is like pure unsweetened white chocolate, which, on its own, has a subtle flavour. It is at melting point that it is absolutely divine and exquisite aroma and flavours are unleashed. Add pure Cacao butter to any of your favourite hot beverages for instant gourmet decadence. Try it in your coffee, maccha, or hot cocoa for an intensely luxurious experience.

The Magic of Cacao Butter—Why Chocolate Melts in Your Hand and Mouth Differently

"Chemically speaking, what makes chocolate so unique and irresistible is that its melting point is slightly below body temperature. Hold a chocolate bar in the palm of your hand and it becomes a gooey mess. But place it on your tongue and, instantly, you're overwhelmed with mouthwatering delight. That's because the Cocoa Butter dissolves first and distributes the rest of the chocolate ingredients over the taste buds in quick succession, starting with sugar. Remove the Cocoa Butter and the entire experience is altered."

Excerpt from the book *The Emperors of Chocolate* by Joel Glenn Brenner

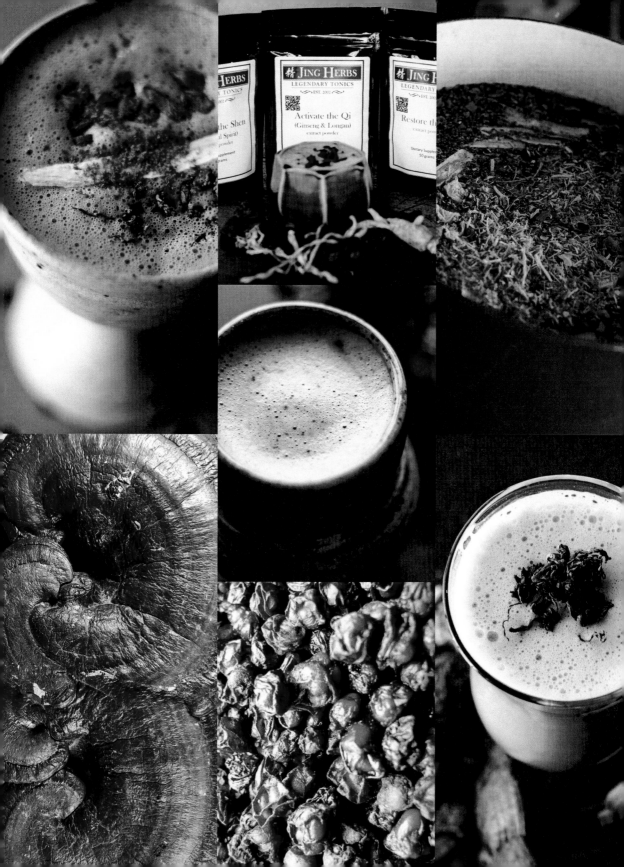

JING HERBS
LEGENDARY TONICS

Activate the Qi
(Ginseng & Longan)
extract powder

Restore the

Three Treasures Elixirs

—————— Craft Your Own Nourishing Beverages ——————

THREE TREASURES TONIC
Reishi, Cordyceps

AWAKEN THE SHEN

RESTORE THE JING

ACTIVATE THE QI

ELIXIR OF LONGEVITY
Goji

Tao (pronounced Dow), is a Chinese word meaning 'way' and 'path'. As well, it is a 'doctrine' or 'principle'. Chinese tonic herbalism is derived from the Taoist traditions in China.

According to Taoist tradition, there are three fundamental energies housed in all living beings: Essence (Jing), Energy (Qi), and Spirit (Shen). The integration of these three energies constitutes our very existence, and they are considered to be treasures to be protected, nourished, and balanced.

It has been perceived that certain herbs contain the qualities of these fundamental energies and, by consuming them, one can help protect, nourish, and balance these qualities within. We have designed these Elixirs based upon this philosophy, and are using formulas designed with the expertise of Dr. George Lamoureaux from Jing Herbs.

The Elixirs are Restore the Jing, Awaken the Shen, and Activate the Qi. Each carefully designed formula contains anywhere from eight to thirteen key and supportive herbs—these are the real stars in these Elixirs.

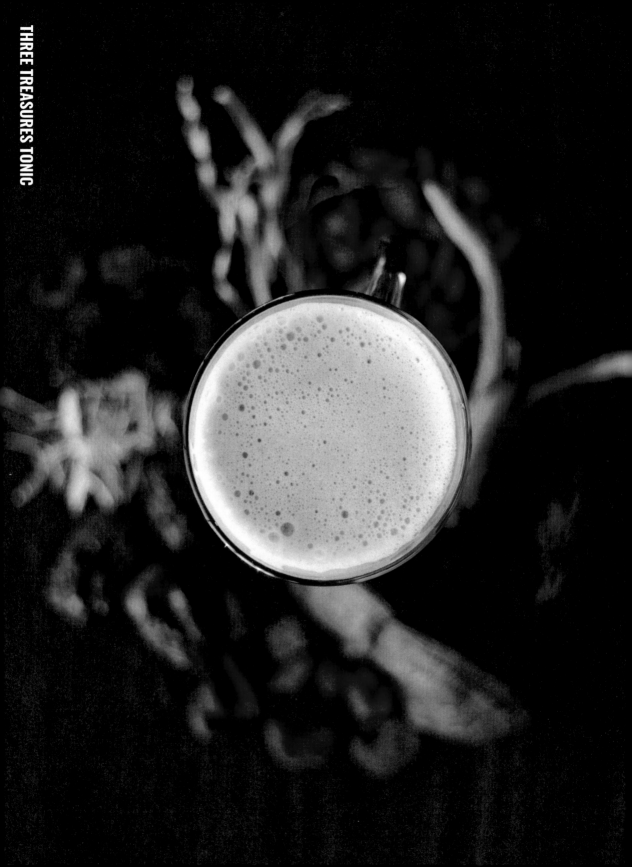

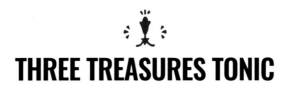

THREE TREASURES TONIC

May your energies be nourished, protected, and balanced. A potent of blend of all Three Treasures in one Elixir.

INGREDIENTS

12 ounces of brewed Reishi tea

½ teaspoon Restore the Jing

½ teaspoon Awaken the Shen

½ teaspoon Activate the Qi

¼ teaspoon Chaga extract

¼ teaspoon Reishi extract

¼ teaspoon Cordyceps extract

2 teaspoons Honey

2 teaspoons Lucuma

1 Tablespoon Coconut butter

¼ teaspoon Vanilla

pinch of your choice high-quality salt

METHOD

Blend all on high with half the tea. Pour into desired cup and fill the rest of the way with remaining hot Reishi tea.

UPGRADE

½ teaspoon He Shou Wu powder

REISHI *Ganoderma lucidum*

Reishi's name, Ganoderma, means shiny skin. It is derived from gano, meaning shiny, and derma, meaning skin. It's commonly known as the 'Varnished Conk' for its glossy, almost shellacked-looking exterior. Many types of Ganoderma grow throughout the world; it comes in a variety of colours including red, black, brown, and purple—although Red Reishi seems to be the most common and notable.

Reishi mushroom, with its multiple variations and aliases, has been used for over 2000 years to fight symptoms of aging, which is why it has been given the name: the Mushroom of Immortality. Reishi benefits the body's organs and systems, including helping the immune system, providing liver protection, and assisting the cardiovascular system. Reishi is host to a unique and dynamic array of organic compounds which include triterpenes, alkaloids, sterols, and various essential polysaccharides, which are long-chain sugars that feed the immune system. Its benefits include anti-aging, stress-relieving, immune-modulating, antioxidant, blood pressure stabilization, neuroprotective effects, and anti-inflammatory properties.

"Taoists continuously claimed that Reishi promotes calmness, centeredness, balance, inner awareness and inner strength.

...Reishi was believed to help calm the mind, ease tension, strengthen the nerves, strengthen memory, sharpen concentration, improve focus, build willpower and as a result, help build wisdom. That is why it is called 'The Herb of Spiritual Potency'." Ron Teeguarden on Duanwood Reishi.

CORDYCEPS *Cordyceps sinensis*

Known as the 'caterpillar fungus' in China, Cordyceps are a unique and rare relationship between insect and fungus. Because of its rarity, Cordyceps were originally reserved for the use of the Emperor and his royal family in ancient China. Today, Cordyceps is a medicinal mushroom that has earned a reputation for increasing athletic performance, as well serving as a superior libido enhancer for men and women. It is a vitalizing, anti-stress Qi tonic that can restore the deep-energy depleted by stress. It is also a valuable lung tonic, and is used to strengthen the respiratory system. Cordyceps mushrooms can be found and used in whole, powdered, or extract form. Any, or all, are awesome for adding to your Elixirs.

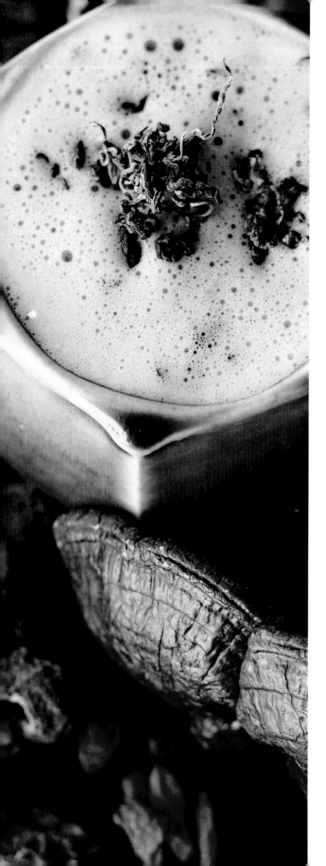

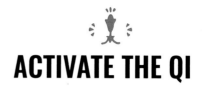

ACTIVATE THE QI

An Elixir to uplift your energy, while easing stress.

INGREDIENTS

12 ounces of brewed Reishi tea

1 teaspoon Activate the Qi

¼ teaspoon Cordyceps extract

1 teaspoon Honey

2 teaspoon Lucuma

½ teaspoon Ginger powder

2 drops Ginger essential oil

1 Tablespoon Coconut butter

pinch of your choice high-quality salt

METHOD

Blend ingredients on high with half the tea. Pour into desired cup and fill the rest of the way with hot Reishi tea.

UPGRADE

¼ teaspoon Ashwaganda

ACTIVATE THE QI is a herbal formula that from the company Jing Herbs. Ginseng & Longan are the main herbs in this formula that can offer energy during the day and help you fall asleep at night. These herbs are known to strengthen digestion, support the building of blood, and have a calming effect on the emotions.

Activate the Qi Blend: 10:1 extracts of Atractylodes rhizome, Jujube seed, Longan fruit, Astragalus root, Poria sclerotium, Panax Ginseng root, Dong Quai root, Ginger, Saussurea costus root, red jujube fruit, Polygala root, Chinese licorice root

· · · · · · · · ·

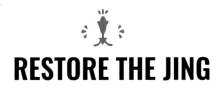

RESTORE THE JING

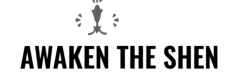

AWAKEN THE SHEN

A restorative Elixir to replenish and revitalize core energy of the body - Jing Essence.

An elixir to nurture the heart and cultivate a peaceful spirit.

INGREDIENTS

12 ounces of brewed Reishi tea

1 teaspoon Restore the Jing

¼ teaspoon Chaga extract

1 teaspoon Honey

2 teaspoon Lucuma

1 Tablespoon Coconut butter

⅛ teaspoon Cardamom powder

2 drops Bergamot essential oil

pinch of your choice high-quality salt

METHOD

Blend ingredients on high with half the tea. Pour into desired cup and fill the rest of the way with hot Reishi tea.

UPGRADE

Up the Anti:
¼ teaspoon He Shou Wu

RESTORE THE JING is a herbal formula from

the company Jing Herbs. It combines the power of two tonic herbs, Eucommia and Morinda, and the restorative attributes of the other supportive herbs to create a perfectly balanced longevity tonic to replenish and vitalize the core energy of the body, your Jing Essence.

Restore the Jing Blend: 10:1 extracts of Eucommia bark, Morinda root, Rhemannia root, Cornus fruit, Dioscorea rhizome (Chinese Yam), Poria sclerotium, Alisma rhizome, Moutan root bark

INGREDIENTS

12 ounces of brewed Reishi tea

1 teaspoon Awaken the Shen

¼ teaspoon Reishi extract

1 Tablespoon Honey

2 teaspoons Lucuma

1 Tablespoon Coconut butter

½ teaspoon Cinnamon

1 drop Cinnamon bark oil

pinch of your choice high-quality salt

METHOD

Blend ingredients on high with half the tea. Pour into desired cup and fill the rest of the way with hot Reishi tea.

UPGRADE

¼ teaspoon Pearl Powder

AWAKEN THE SHEN is a herbal formula

from the company Jing Herbs. The chief herbs, Reishi, Albizia, Asparagus, and Polygala together are said to put a smile on your face and melt your worries away. Let your spirit soar and your dreams come true as you connect to your divine energy and cultivate happiness on a moment-to-moment basis.

Awaken the Shen Blend: 10:1 extracts of Reishi fruiting body, Albizia flower, Chinese Asparagus root, Polygala root, Pearl powder, Longan fruit, Spirit Poria sclerotium, Eclipta herb, Chinese Salvia root, He Shou Wu, Bupleurum root, White peony root, Schizandra fruit

ELIXIR OF LONGEVITY

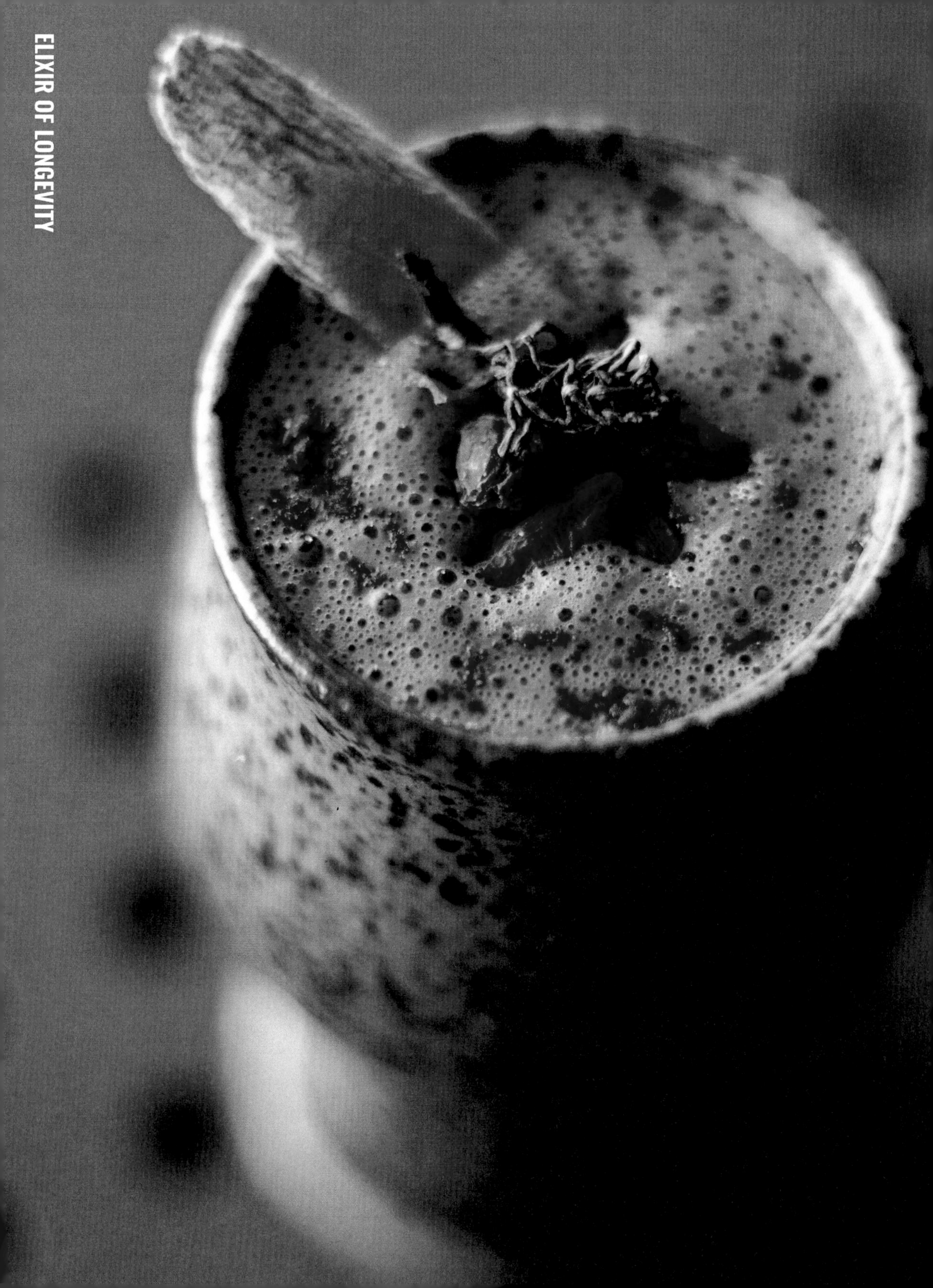

ELIXIR OF LONGEVITY

An herbal blessing from the five ancient immortals of Chinese herbalism for a long, healthy life.

INGREDIENTS

12 ounces brewed Gynostemma tea

1 Tablespoon Coconut butter

1 Tablespoon Goji berries

1 Tablespoon Dandy Blend

1 Tablespoon Honey

½ teaspoon He Shou Wu

½ teaspoon Astragalus powder

½ teaspoon Schizandra powder

METHOD

Blend ingredients on high with half the tea. Pour into desired cup and fill the rest with the remaining hot tea.

GOJI BERRY *Lycium barbarum*

In Asia, Goji has been eaten for centuries by those with hopes to lengthen life.

Known as the 'Fountain of Youth', this ancient, medicinal fruit is an amazing source of antioxidants, particularly carotenoids—that is, beta-carotene and zeaxanthin which are excellent for, and protective to, the eyes.

Packed with essential amino acids, Goji is rare amongst berries for being a complete protein.

Goji has been used to treat many common ailments such as diabetes, high blood pressure, and age-related eye problems.

Traditionally, when consumed, Goji berries were often cooked in soups or rice congees, as well as used for herbal teas.

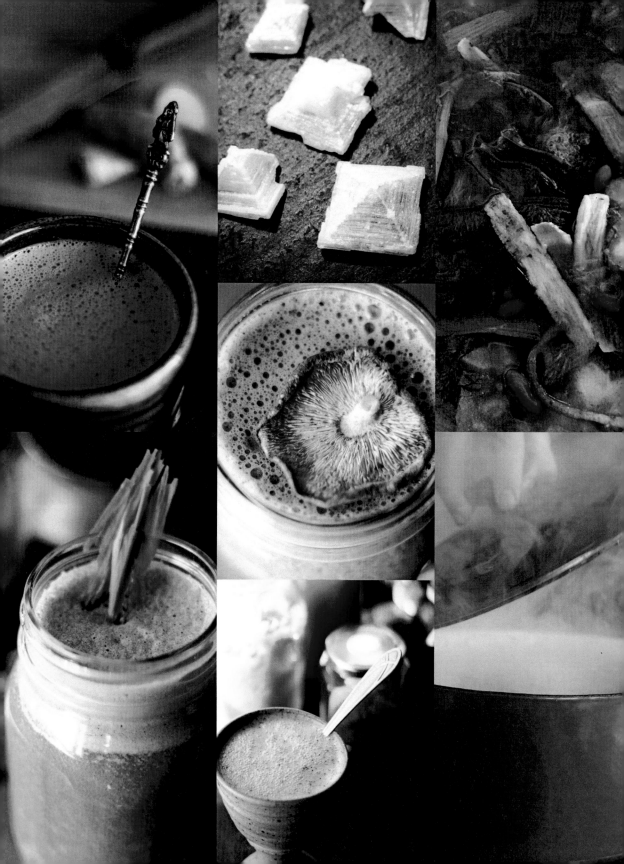

Savoury Elixirs

Craft Your Own Nourishing Beverages

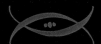

**BONE BROTH &
MEAT STOCK**

MISO HAPPY
Tocotrienols

4 KINGDOMS
Turkey Tail

FOREST MUSHROOM
Lion's Mane

CURRY OM
Miso

Savoury Elixirs are gaining momentum; the trend of bone broth drinks and the concept of Elixirs has come together.

We have crafted various savoury Elixirs in a few ways. One contains bone broth as a base but you can make each with a base of herbal tea, vegetable broth, bone broth, or meat stock.

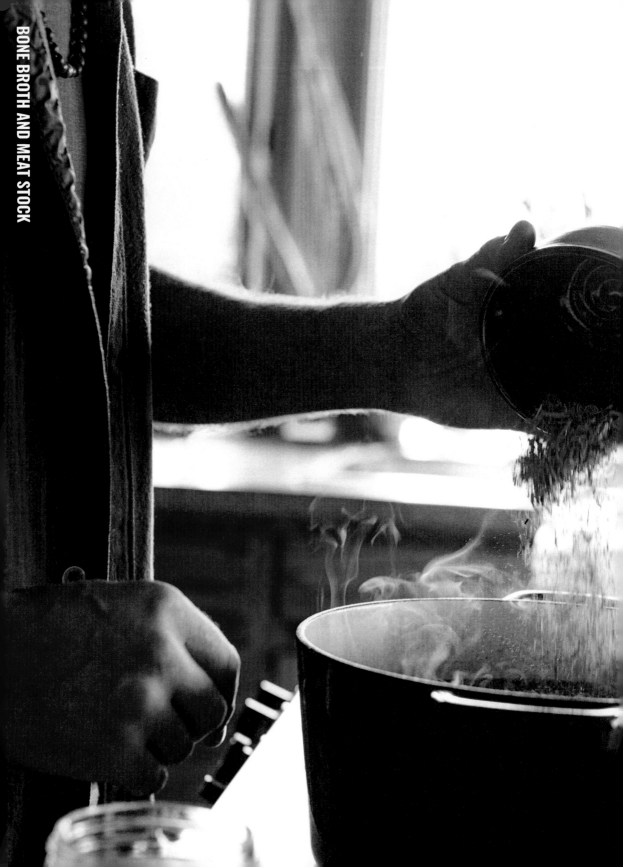

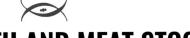

BONE BROTH AND MEAT STOCK

Nutrient rich bases for your Savoury Elixirs.

INGREDIENTS

Water

Bones

Culinary herbs

Vegetables

Tonic herbs

Medicinal Mushrooms

Sea Vegetables

Vinegar

BONE BROTH

It's easy to prepare deeply nourishing bone broth. It's also a great way to use scraps. Bone broth adds flavour and nutrients to Elixirs in a wonderful umami way. Included is a list of key ingredients I add to almost every bone broth I make. You can add them all (or not), to your base of bones and water. Pick and choose for variety. Use what you have on hand. Decide your desired amount.

To a large pot of water, add the bones and vinegar first, and then begin to add the other ingredients. The bones can be purchased fresh, or you can use those saved from a meal. I recommend adding collagen-rich feet or hooves from various animals. This increases nutrient density and offers delicious jellying properties.

Once all ingredients are in the pot, turn the heat to high until the water reaches a simmer, then turn to low and simmer from TWO to TWENTY-FOUR hours to fully extract all of the goodness. When the broth is done, strain and jar. I like to keep enough in the fridge (to use over the next few days). Freeze the rest so there's always a supply on hand for Elixir making and other cooking.

INGREDIENTS

Water

Bones

Meat

Culinary herbs

Vegetables

Tonic herbs

Medicinal Mushrooms

Sea Vegetables

Vinegar

MEAT STOCK

Meat Stock is similar to creating bone broth, but meat is included along with the bones. This can be meat on a bone, or a whole chicken. It is highly recommended to add chicken or duck feet as well. I have also come to enjoy adding organ meats to meat stock. It's another way to get valuable foods into my family's diet—especially when the flavour of the organ meats, on their own, is not always appreciated. One key difference between meat stock and bone broth is that meat stock is simmered for a short amount of time for around ninety minutes and up to three hours (still at a low temperature). This retains key nutrients like glutamine, essential for healing the gut.

Bone broth or meat stock? Which should you consume?

In short, if you have any kind of digestive distress, acute or chronic, then meat stock is the way to go. It has been shown to help heal and seal the gut. If there are no gut issues, or after gut issues are resolved, enjoy either.

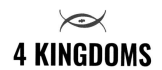

4 KINGDOMS

INGREDIENTS

8 ounces of warm bone broth or meat stock

2 Tablespoons Miso

½ to 1 teaspoon hot sauce (depending on desired spiciness)

1 Tablespoon grass-fed butter or ghee

¼ teaspoon Cajun spice seasoning mix (or other seasoning blends, like Curry powder)

¼ teaspoon Medicinal Mushroom extract powder. Either a blend of many different mushrooms, or a single medicinal mushroom, like Turkey Tail.

METHOD

Bring all ingredients together in a blender. Blend on high, pour into a tall mug or jar, and enjoy.

This recipe is an absolute revelation. I had been consuming the sweeter, earthy, and even dark, bitter Elixirs for a couple years before I was introduced to the idea of a savoury Elixir.

It was my friend and colleague, Daniel Vitalis, who introduced me to the concept of using a bone broth as the base for an Elixir, with Miso, butter, and hot sauce for the flavour. Daniel has always been an innovator in the field of natural health, helping many move forward with greater clarity. He and I share the view of the 4 'Kingdoms' of life as an ideal and helpful approach to whole food, natural nutrition. These 4 Kingdom Food Groups are: Plants, Animals, Bacteria, and Fungi.

This Elixir brings the unique nutrition offered by each of the 4 Kingdoms. A delicious combination.

TURKEY TAIL *Coriolus or Trametes versicolour*

Chinese legend is filled with stories of those who discovered this mushroom and became immortal.

One of the most well studied mushrooms in the world, Turkey Tail takes centre stage, demonstrating immune modulating properties that help those who are healthy, and assist those dealing with chronic disease. Associated with longevity, health, and spiritual attunement, the Turkey Tail mushroom is said to be beneficial for one's spirit and vital energy. Its scope of immune enhancing properties includes its use to treat infections, inflammation, and general immune system weakness.

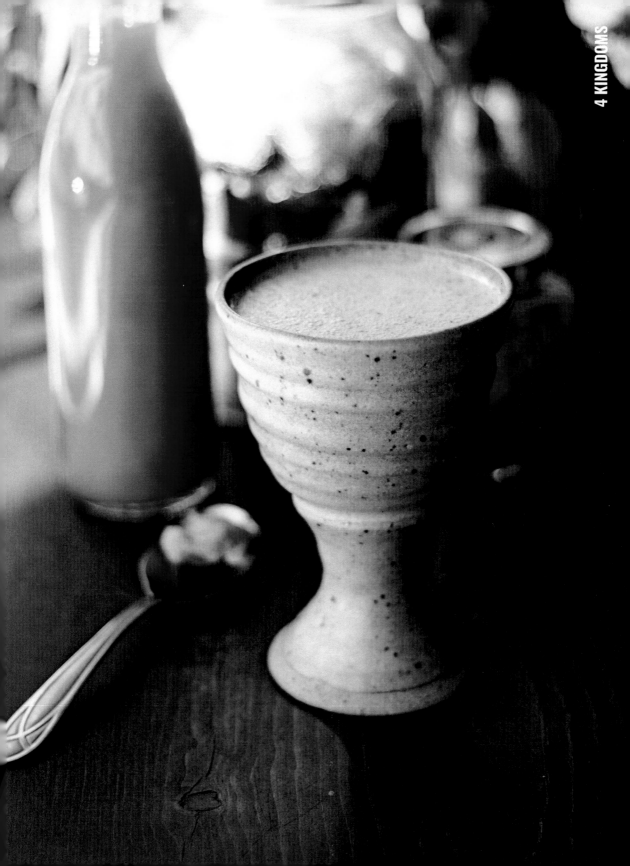

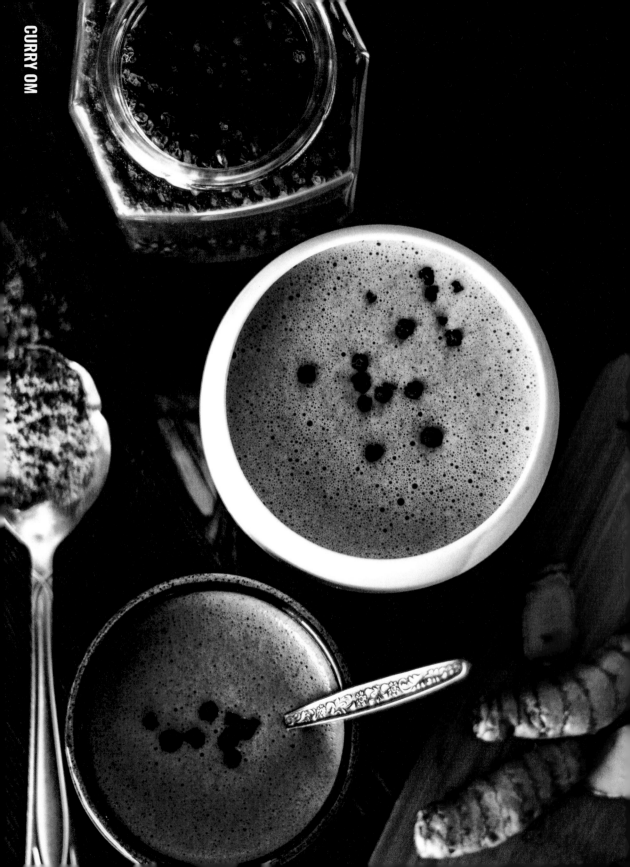

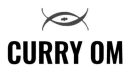

CURRY OM

A deep, warming experience, perfectly sour and spicy, and completely delicious.

INGREDIENTS

12 ounces of hot Reishi tea

1 Tablespoon Miso

1 Tablespoon Coconut butter

1 Tablespoon Sour cherries - optional

3 sun-dried Tomato halves cut into pieces – optional

2 teaspoons Curry powder

1 teaspoon Nutritional Yeast

1 teaspoon Moringa powder

½ teaspoon Cumin powder

½ teaspoon Cardamom powder

Cayenne pepper to taste

METHOD

Blend ingredients together with half of the tea, then top up with the rest of the hot Reishi tea.

UPGRADE

1 teaspoon Collagen Peptides

MISO

According to Japanese folklore, Miso is 'a gift from the gods to ensure health and longevity'.

Miso is a dense vegetarian protein which is permanently preserved through the perfect proliferation of probiotics.

This fermented paste is made from the spores of a fungus called Koji, Aspergillus oryzae. Typically a fermented rice and bean combination, though often just beans (such as soy), Miso has been consumed for centuries with hundreds of regional and cultural variations. It provides an instant flavour foundation to any dish, dressing, or drink, adding what's been described as the fifth flavour: umami.

It is rich in vitamins and minerals, including lots of B vitamins and folic acid. When purchasing Miso, look for unpasteurized, live, enzyme-rich products that need to be stored in the fridge.

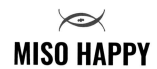

MISO HAPPY

This warming soup is green and alkalizing. It contains the nourishing qualities
of Kelp, Chlorella, Miso and Shiitake mushroom.

INGREDIENTS

12 ounces of hot Reishi tea

2 Tablespoons Miso

1 teaspoon Chlorella

1½ teaspoon Ginger powder

⅛ teaspoon Kelp powder

1 Tablespoon Tahini

2 teaspoons Tocotrienols

1½ teaspoons Shiitake powder

METHOD

Blend with half of the tea, then
top up with the rest of the hot
Reishi tea.

UPGRADE

1 teaspoon Collagen Peptides

TOCOTRIENOLS

Tocotrienols are compounds that are members of the vitamin E family.
The name is given to a preparation of raw rice bran powder that is a
concentrated source of bioavailable Tocotrienols. Few people realize
that vitamin E is a family of eight different compounds, of which there
are four Tocotrienols and four Tocopherols. Most vitamin E sold as a
supplement is sold as Alpha Tocopherol, which is good, but represents
only one of the eight compounds.

Vitamin E is known as being a great antioxidant, valued for heart health
and protection, skin and hair lustre, brain and nervous system health,
lowering blood pressure, and reducing cholesterol.

Tocotrienols rice bran is naturally gluten-free, and provides a mildly
sweet, and a luxuriously creamy taste, that melts in your mouth.
Perfect for Elixirs.

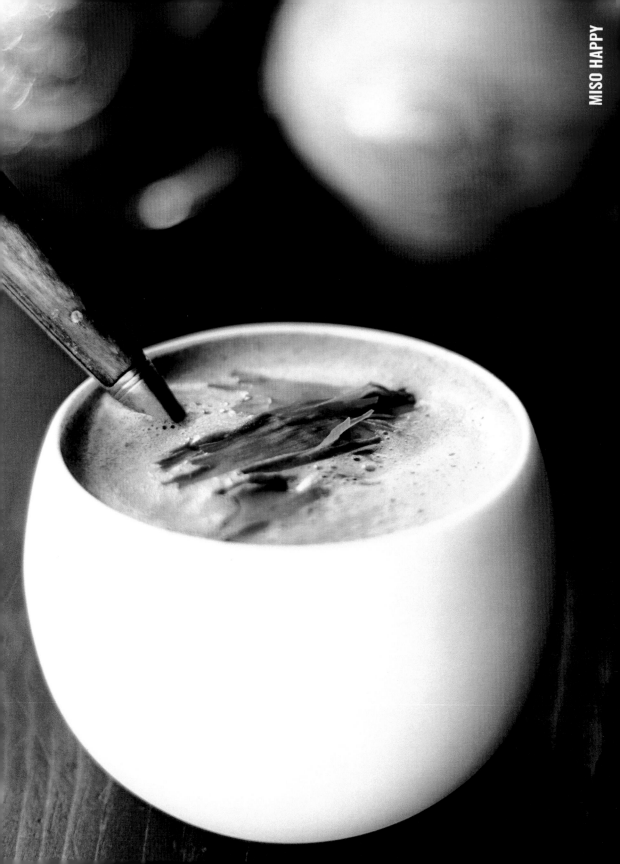

FOREST MUSHROOM

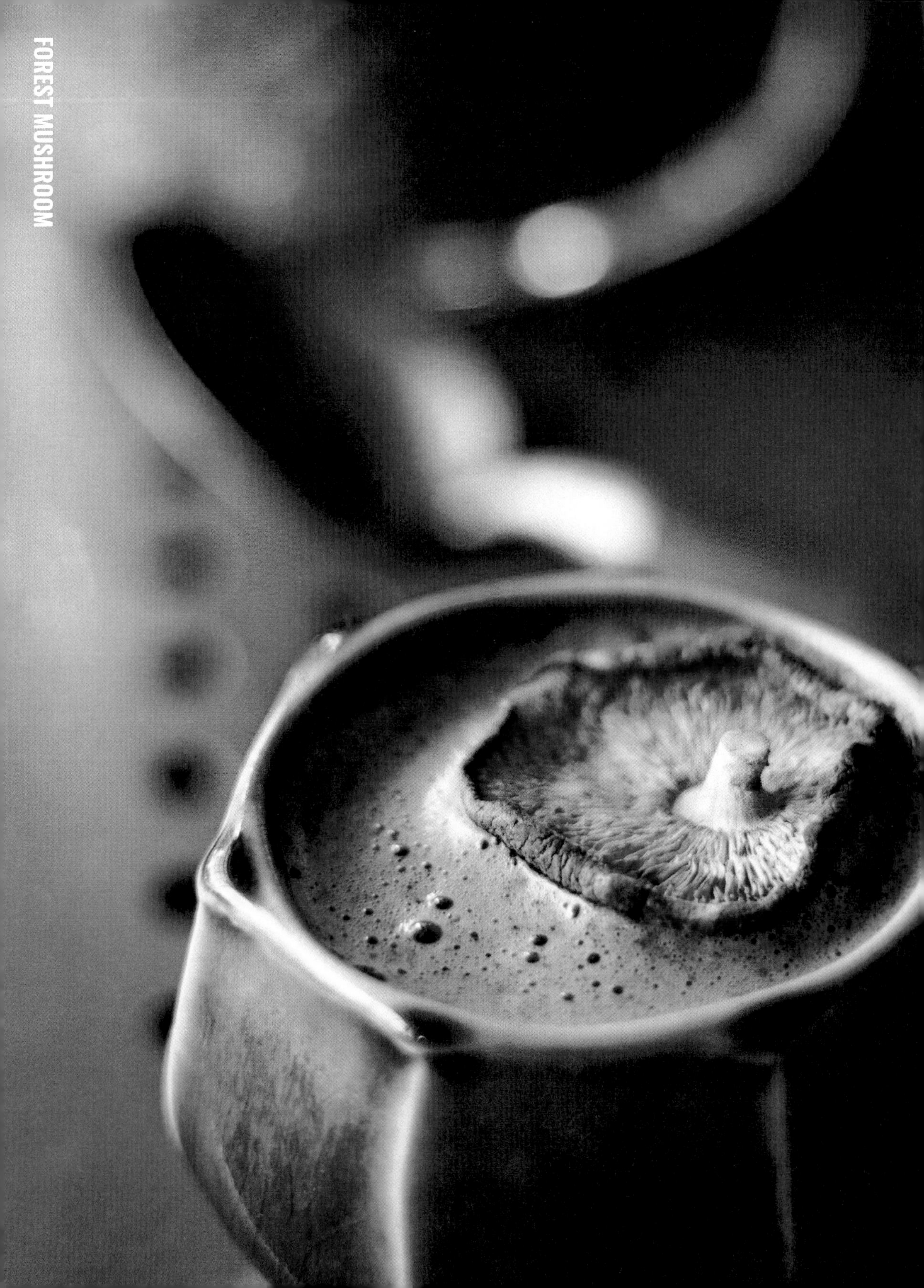

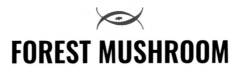

FOREST MUSHROOM

A superfood spin on an earthy classic.

INGREDIENTS

6 ounces brewed Chaga tea

6 ounces brewed Reishi tea

1 Tablespoon Coconut butter

1 Tablespoon Miso

1 Tablespoon Tocotrienols

1 Tablespoon Olive oil

1 teaspoon Maple syrup

1 teaspoon Medicinal Mushroom blend powder

½ teaspoon Maca powder

½ teaspoon Mesquite powder

½ teaspoon Maitake or Lion's Mane mushroom powder

½ teaspoon Winter Savoury

¼ teaspoon Thyme

⅛ teaspoon Garlic powder

1 pinch Himalayan salt

METHOD

Blend on high with half the tea. Pour into desired cup and fill the rest of the way with hot Chaga tea.

UPGRADE

1 teaspoon Collagen Peptides
1 Tablespoon Colostrum
2 teaspoons Ghee

LION'S MANE *Hericium erinacae*

This medicinal mushroom is claimed to be a food that enhances memory and mood. It is heralded for its unparalleled benefits for the brain and nervous system, primarily due to it containing Nerve Growth Factor (NGF). Research shows it improves cognitive function, helps with nerve regeneration, improves digestive function, and is immuno-supportive, anti-inflammatory, and an antioxidant. Lion's Mane and other mushrooms in the Hericium genus are delicious culinary and medicinal mushrooms that can be consumed whole, as a meal, or for Elixirs, will be in powdered and extract form.

For more information about Medicinal Mushrooms check out the book by Robert Rogers (RH) AHG *The Fungal Pharmacy: The Complete Guide to Medicinal Mushrooms & Lichens of North America*

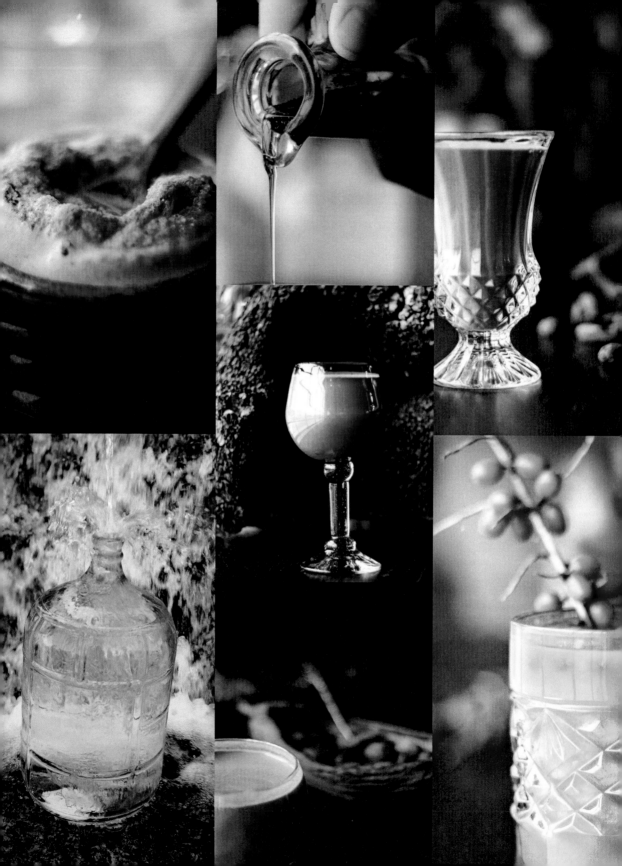

Chilled Elixirs

—— Craft Your Own Nourishing Beverages ——

SOLAR CHARGE
Seabuckthorn, Camu Camu

CHAGA ICED CAPPUCCINO
Chaga

CHAGA CHOCOLATE MYLKSHAKE
Cacao

ROOT BEER
Classic Herbs of Root Beer

ICED MACCHA LATTE
Maccha

Not all Elixirs need to be made and consumed warm. You can craft cooling and refreshing creations applying the same principles of Elixir making. Enjoy the diversity offered by temperature.

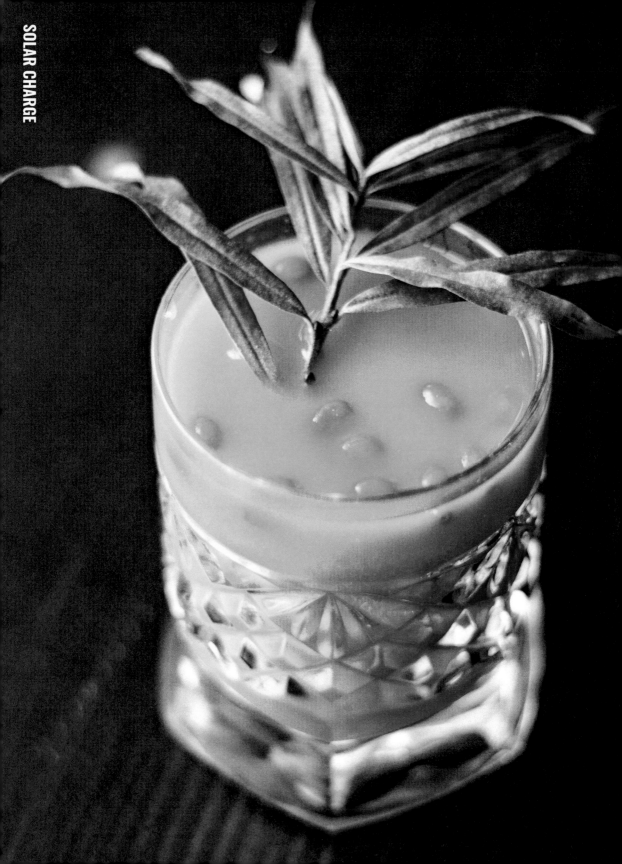

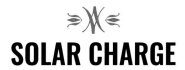

SOLAR CHARGE

Equals walking on sunshine.

INGREDIENTS

½ cup of 'Solberry'
Seabuckthorn puree

1½ Tablespoons Camu Camu
powder

½ cup raw unheated Honey

4 drops high-quality orange or
tangerine essential oil

4 cups Spring water
(approx. one litre)

METHOD

Blend and enjoy with gratitude
and positive intentions.

UPGRADE

1 teaspoon Schizandra extract

This Elixir is delightfully bright and refreshing. It's a great pick-me-up any time, and a good go-to if you're coming down with something or already under the weather.

This recipe makes 5 cups or just over one litre of pure sunshine in a bottle. Its goodness can be consumed throughout your day or stored in the fridge for a week.

SEABUCKTHORN *Hippophae rhamnoides*

The most common of seven species, Seabuckthorn is a superfruit full of omegas 3, 6, 9, and 7, whose powers go more than skin deep; it's responsible for a natural, healthy glow. It's been used for centuries, for nourishment and healing, within many cultures. In folk medicine, it was known as 'Life Oil' or 'God Sent Medicine'. The mythical Pegasus is said to have eaten the berries to gain the power to fly.

Seabuckthorn contains over 190 phytonutrients including the antioxidants Superoxide dismutase and Vitamin C to fight free-radicals.

An incredibly hardy bush, its extensive root system is capable of fixing nitrogen. Beyond its food value, it's a giver and sharer, its life cycle helping fertilize soil and making good bacteria available for other plants.

It is said that the leaves and branches were fed as a supplement to horses to support health and give a shiny appearance of the coat, hence the reference in its Latin name hippo (horse) and phaos (shining).

CAMU CAMU *Myrcriaria dubia*

Camu Camu is a superfruit containing the highest amount of Vitamin C of any fruit, it has been found to contain 1000—3000 milligrams of Vitamin C per 100 grams of fresh pulp which is 60 times more than Oranges. Staggeringly, ONE teaspoon of dried Camu powder provides more than 600% of the RDA (recommended daily allowance) of Vitamin C. And, that's whole-food form, not just Ascorbic acid. Beyond Vitamin C, Camu Camu comes with a host of other amazing compounds and benefits, and has been used for myriad solutions: inflammation, eye and gut health, boosting the immune system, and improving mood.

CHAGA CHOCOLATE MYLKSHAKE

Creamy, Divine Chocolate Delight.

INGREDIENTS

1 cup cold Chaga tea or Spring water with 1 teaspoon Chaga extract

¼ cup raw Cashews (soaked)

1 Tablespoon Lucuma

1½ Tablespoons Cacao powder

1½ Tablespoons Coconut Palm sugar

½ teaspoon Vanilla extract or powder

METHOD

Blend with love. Consume with passion.

Wonderful served chilled. Equally delicious when warmed.

UPGRADE

Raw Cow or Goat milk as a base instead of Cashew milk

Once upon a Chaga Chocolate Mylkshake... we unveiled this Elixir at a live event with over 2000 attendees; and our booth had the longest line-up — dozens and dozens of people willing to wait to taste.

The creaminess is a result of soaking the Cashews and blending them in a high-speed blender—they do not need straining as other nut mylks do. The moist Cashews dissolve leaving a full-bodied creaminess that is added to by the Lucuma.

Though the feature foods are Cacao and Chaga, all the other ingredients play more than a supporting role.

CACAO AKA CHOCOLATE *Theobroma cacao*

Chocolate, one of the most delicious, sensual, and magical foods.

One of the few foods that can create love at first bite...

Think of Theobroma Cacao as the love child of Willy Wonka and a stunning Earth goddess; she is delicious, energetic, and funny, yet exquisitely divine.

Cacao beans are chocolate. 100%. You cannot have chocolate without cacao.

Cacao is the nut or seed of the chocolate tree, Theobroma cacao, which literally translates as 'Food of the Gods'.

Cacao can be processed into many forms including beans, nibs, paste, powder, and butter, all of which then can be transformed into myriad delectable dishes that can be sweet, bitter, savoury, or spicy. Here in the context of a cold Elixir, I have used cacao powder as an easy way to bring the rich chocolate goodness to this drink. I recommend using only cacao powder that has not been dutched. The dutch-processing of cacao drastically reduces the nutritional and energetic potency.

When Elixir crafting, you can add cacao (as beans, nibs, paste, powder and/or butter) to bring deep chocolaty flavours and feelings to any drink.

WITH CACAO, YOU'RE IN THE NOW

Cacao is one of my top productivity tools for enhancing focus and creativity. It can absolutely land you in the zone.

Cacao flavanols have been shown to improve cognitive function, help with memory retention, and increase processing speed and information recall.

Though cacao does contain a small amount of caffeine, a known brain stimulant, the level is a fraction of that in a cup of coffee. In essence, this small amount adds in the synergy of creating energy and helps with clear thinking.

ANADAMIDE - CHOCOLATE BLISS

Cacao also contains Anandamide, a neurotransmitter which synthesizes in the body and fits into the THC receptor sites of the brain. Anandamide is known as the bliss molecule. Cacao contains this AND the compounds that inhibit the breakdown of anandamide.

Anandamide exhibits anti-anxiety and antidepressant properties... and then goes one step further. Research has shown that Anandamide positively affects areas of the brain which are important in memory, motivation, and higher thought process.

And it's not just Anandamide; cacao also delivers a boost of neurotransmitters like dopamine and serotonin which are both feel-good brain chemicals. Cacao also contains tryptophan, an amino acid that plays an important role in the synthesis of the neurotransmitter: serotonin. Serotonin is associated with feelings of well-being.

By now, I'm sure you're beginning to see the validation for your love-affair with chocolate—a focus-fuelled tool, a creative enhancer, and one of the best antidepressants.

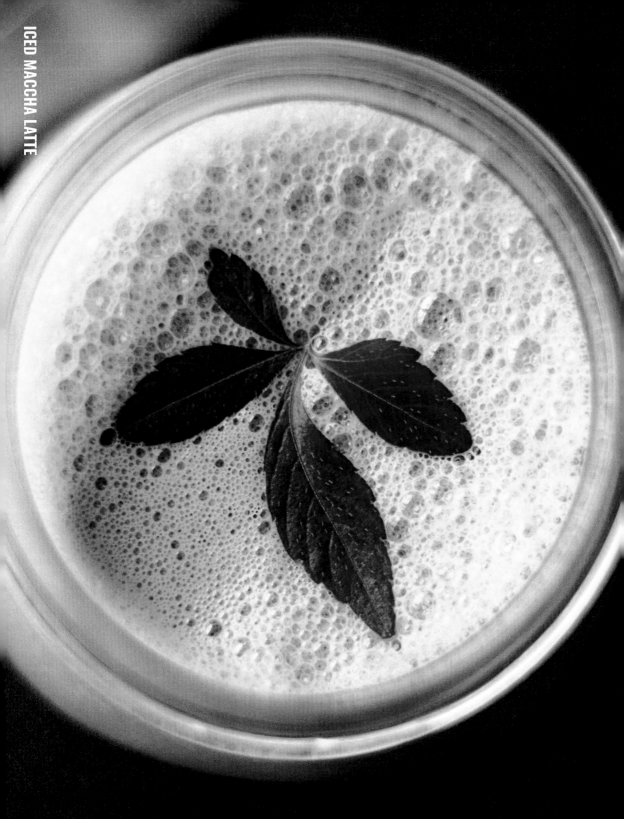

ICED MACCHA LATTE

Cooling, refreshing, and naturally uplifting. Simplicity in the creation of refreshing clean, green energy.

INGREDIENTS

⅓ cup of room-temperature Gynostemma, Nettle, Peppermint, or any favourite herbal tea

1 Tablespoon Lucuma

1 Tablespoon Honey or your choice and amount of sweetener

¼ teaspoon Vanilla

2 drops Jasmine oil and/or 1 drop Lemon oil, Peppermint, or Ginger (optional)

2 teaspoons Coconut oil - can be switched for organic butter

1 teaspoon Maccha powder

8 ounces of ice

METHOD

Blend all ingredients together, except the ice. Once well combined add ice and finish blending.

MACCHA *Camellia sinensis*

Maccha or Matcha tea is made by harvesting only the tips of the leaves of a specially grown green tea, Camellia sinensis.

Just like fine wine requires the best grapes, or delectable chocolate requires the purest Cacao, so too does the finest Maccha require superior green tea.

We use the finest of Maccha powder from a company called JagaSilk based out of Victoria, BC. They source their Maccha green tea direct from Mr. Takaki, a farmer in Japan with whom they have a personal relationship. This stellar quality of green tea is from the first flush of leaves, finely stoneground and sealed for freshness. The result is an ultra-fine milled powder that is a bright vibrant green unparalleled color and flavour.

Camellia sinensis contains a key compound called L-Theanine that is known to reduce mental and physical stress, improve cognition, boost mood, and enhance cognitive performance. Additionally, it helps reduce the jitters associated with caffeine intake, since it has a reduced amount of the natural stimulant.

CHAGA ICED CAPPUCCINO

Exhilarating, invigorating, and down-to-earth. A unique twist on a distinguished classic.

INGREDIENTS

12 ounces of steeped Chaga tea

1 Tablespoon Almond butter

1 teaspoon Coconut oil

1 Tablespoon Lucuma

1 Tablespoon Maca powder

2 teaspoons Mesquite powder

1 teaspoon Dandy Blend

1 teaspoon Maple syrup

pinch of your choice
high-quality salt

METHOD

Blend all ingredients with ice

Serve in desired cup with a
spoon and/or straw.

CHAGA *Innonotus obliquus*

Known as the 'King of Medicinal Mushrooms', it contains one of the highest known levels of antioxidants, including SOD or Superoxide dismutase an enzyme group that is known to reduce oxidative stress. Among numerous compounds Chaga has constituents that help boost the immune system, balance blood sugar, normalize cholesterol, and is a great source of minerals (like zinc).

Chaga, when extracted properly, has deep earthy tones and dark vanilla flavours—at the Light Cellar, we thought it a great base for our spin on the classic Iced Cappuccino.

Raw Chaga pieces require brewing into a decoction however Chaga is also available in an extract form as powder or tincture. All forms of Chaga are excellent for Elixirs.

For more information about not only medicinal mushrooms but fungi in general check out the inspiring work of Paul Stamets including his books, *Mycelium Running: How Mushrooms Can Help Save the World* as well as *MycoMedicinals: An Informational Treatise on Mushrooms.*

CHAGA ICED CAPPUCCINO

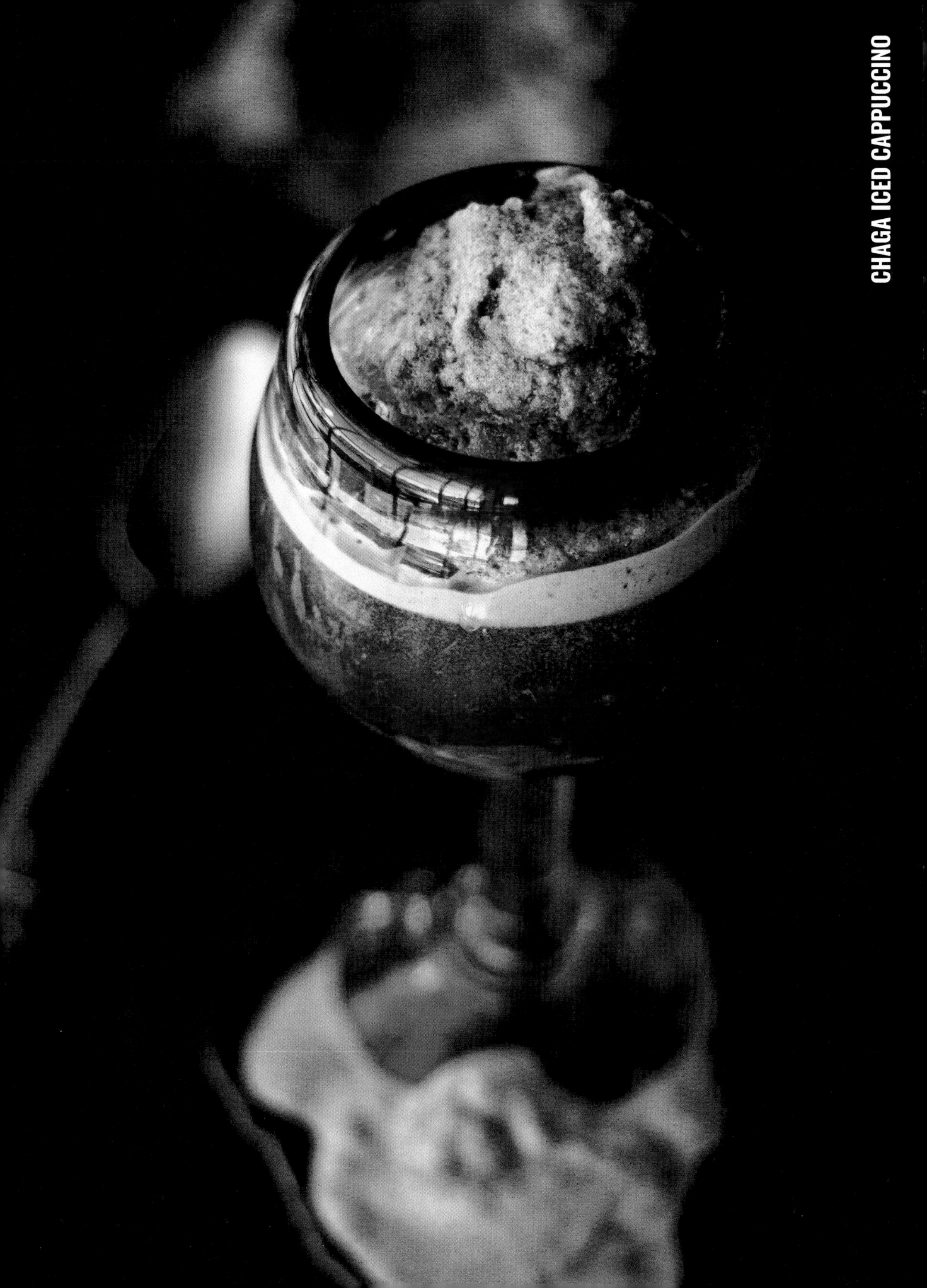

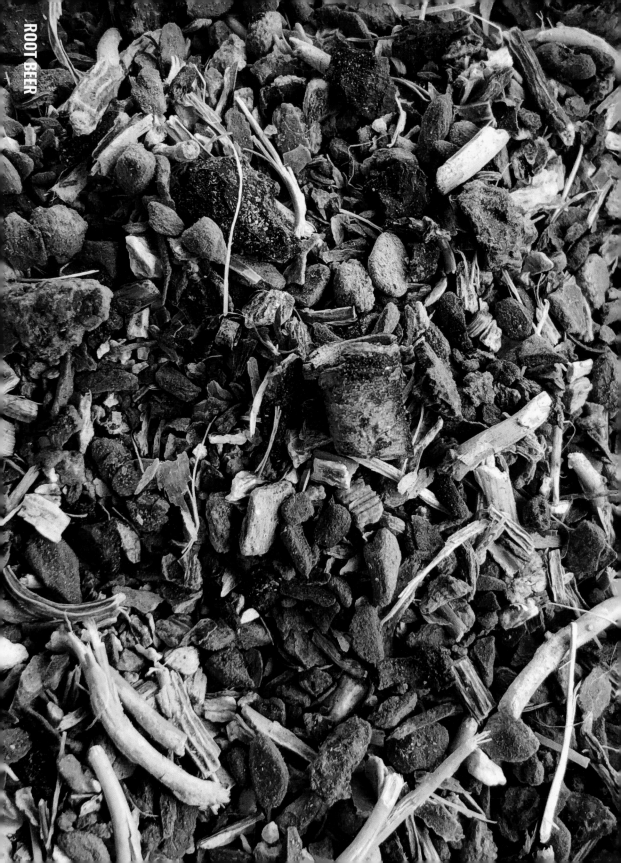

ROOT BEER

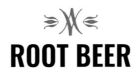

ROOT BEER

Old-fashioned goodness... A liver-loving, blood-cleansing tonic.

METHOD

Bring 4 cups of water to a boil, turn down to a simmer, then add 2-3 Tablespoons of Light Cellar Root Beer tea blend, or any individual 'Root Beer' herbs.

Simmer for at least 10-15 minutes. The longer the simmer, the stronger the tea will be. This can even brew for 1-2 hours with a lid on.

Let cool, sweeten to taste with Maple syrup, dark Cane sugar, Molasses or dark Honey.

This drink will take you back, as you take-back a traditional recipe hijacked by industry and corrupted into a syrupy, slick soda-pop version that dominates convenience store shelves today.

Root Beer has its roots in herbal traditions; this recipe features a number of amazing herbs. Naturally sweetened with a dark maple syrup to perfectly enhance the flavour, your body will savour this drink to the last drop.

This Root Beer Elixir is not carbonated or fermented*. It's simply those familiar flavours in the form of a sweet tea.

There are as many herbs as ways to create Root Beer. From a simple sweetened Sarsaparilla or Sassafras tea to multi-ingredient blends of herbs and spices.

The Light Cellar Root Beer tea blend is created with a base of TEN unique herbs and spices that are synergistically blended to create an iconic flavour and nostalgic taste.

When brewing Root Beer, use our favourite Light Cellar tea blend or pick and choose herbs to which you are drawn. The base of your Root Beer tea should include either: Sassafras or Sarsaparilla.

From that point, add any number of herbs and spices fresh or dried including:

Chaga, un-roasted Dandelion root, Burdock root, Birch bark, Licorice, Spruce, Ginger, Vanilla, Wintergreen, Wild Cherry bark, Allspice, Juniper, Nutmeg, Prickly Ash bark, Yellow dock, Coriander, Hops.

*Traditionally, yeast or a fermentation starter culture was added to naturally create carbonation through fermentation. Today, most root beers are made using syrup concentrate that is force-carbonated with CO2 gas.

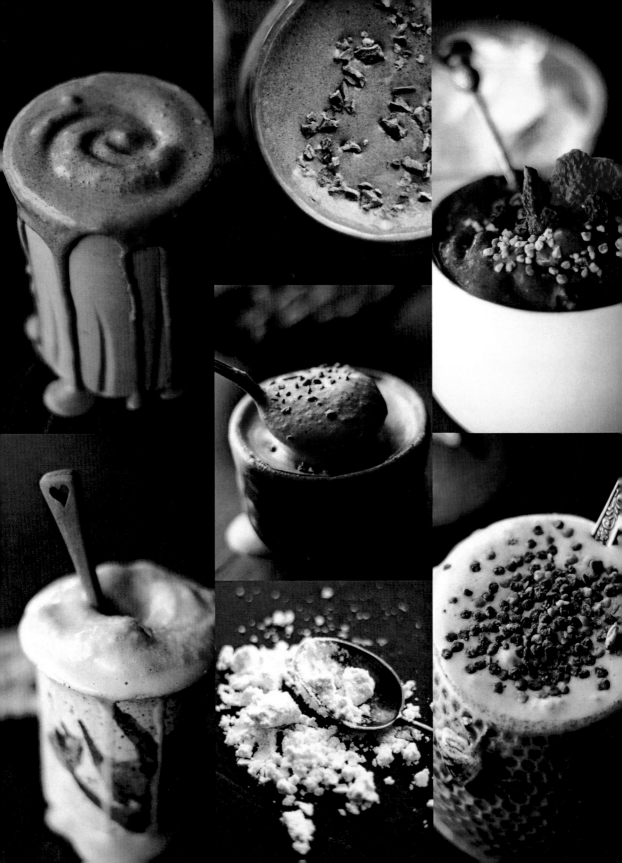

Iced Alchemy

— Craft Your Own Nourishing Beverages —

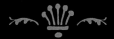

GREEN SPRING	**BERRY SUNRISE**
Spirulina	Baobab
CHOCOLATE STRATOSPHERE	**MYSTIC MOUNTAINTOP**
Whey	Colostrum
EARTH KISS	**GOLDEN HONEYPOT**
Lucuma	Bee foods from the Hive

This is a name Laura and I came up with when we first started making our version of superfood ice creams. They are not quite enough like ice cream to call them such, plus there are regulations as to what is technically an ice cream—for instance 'ice cream' must contain at least 10% milk fat and 20% milk solids. Iced Alchemy is a whole new level above, and a creative twist on, a cold soft-serve delight. They are very popular at our Elixir bar. Each Iced Alchemy will take you a couple minutes to make, which is pretty impressive for any frozen treat made from scratch.

We know you will enjoy these iced Elixirs as much as we do, and see them as more than a treat, rather a meal with powerful herbal and superfood benefits.

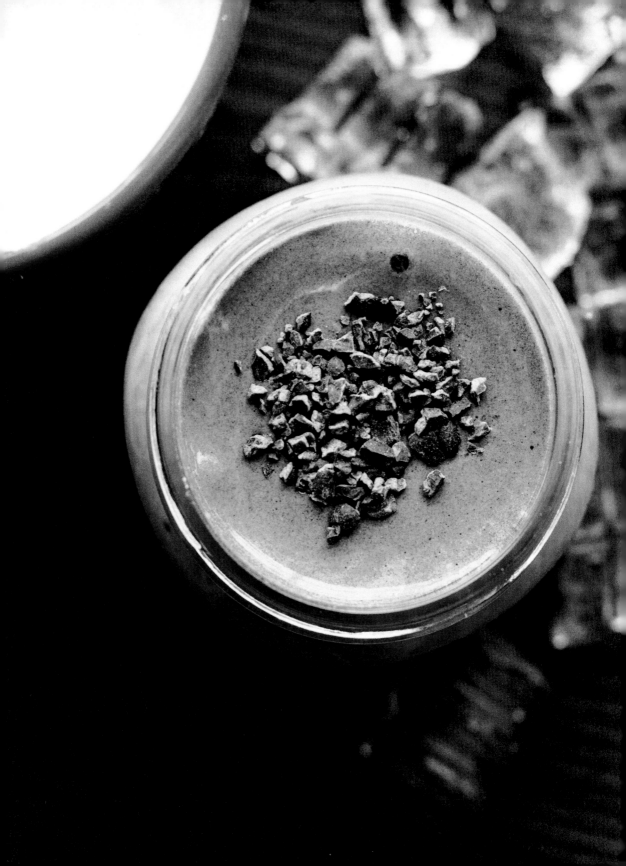

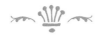

GREEN SPRING

INGREDIENTS

1 Tablespoon Barley Grass powder or Wheat Grass juice powder

1 teaspoon Chlorella or Spirulina powder

2 Tablespoons Lucuma

1 Tablespoon Coconut butter

2 Tablespoons Whey powder

1 Tablespoon Honey

1 Tablespoon Olive oil

¼ teaspoon Himalayan salt

2 drops each of Peppermint oil and Spearmint oil

1 teaspoon Cacao nibs

4 ounces of any cold tea (Gynostemma, Mint, Nettle, Reishi or Chaga...)

12 ounce container of ice (not heaping)

VEGAN

1 Tablespoon Coconut butter

2 Tablespoons of Lucuma

1 Tablespoon Maca

1 Tablespoon Barley Grass or Wheat Grass juice powder

2 teaspoons Chlorella or Spirulina powder

1½ Tablespoons Cane or Palm sugar

1 Tablespoon Olive oil

2 drops each of Peppermint oil and Spearmint Oil

1 Tablespoon Cacao paste

½ teaspoon Vanilla powder

1 Tablespoon Lucuma

½ teaspoon Sunflower or non-GMO Soy lecithin

2 Tablespoons Brown Rice protein powder

4 ounces of any cold tea (Gynostemma, Mint, Nettle, Reishi or Chaga...)

12 ounce container of ice (not heaping)

METHOD

Use a Vitamix blender. Place and combine all dry ingredients except cacao nibs into the blender. Add cold tea and blend until smooth. Add ice and blend again until smooth. Pour into serving vessel. Top with cacao nibs. Enjoy.

SPIRULINA *Arthrospira platensis*

Used for over a thousand years in South America, Spirulina was consumed by Inca and Aztec warriors for endurance and strength.

It is a simple single-celled blue-green algae (cyanobacteria) that grows in a spiral-like shape, hence its name: Spirulina. The word cyan has its roots in a Greek word which means 'blue'.

Some claim Spirulina to be the most nutrient dense food on Earth. Depending on how it is defined and ranked, Spirulina is certainly impressive in what it offers.

Mostly made up of amino acids, including all the essentials, Spirulina is 65% protein delivered in an easy to digest and absorptive form. It is also a rich source of B-complex vitamins known for boosting energy, and for its support for eye, brain, and nerve health. High in iron, to help build blood, especially for vegetarians, as well as containing lots of chlorophyll (the nourishing green pigment that assists in detoxification and removal of toxins), Spirulina contains 26 times the calcium found in milk, and is high in omega 3's, including the anti-inflammatory GLA (Gamma Linolenic Acid).

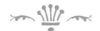

CHOCOLATE STRATOSPHERE

An ecstatic chocolate lift.

INGREDIENTS

3 Tablespoons of cold Chaga tea

1 Tablespoon Coconut butter

3 Tablespoons Whey

2 Tablespoons Lucuma

1 Tablespoon Cacao powder

2 Tablespoons Maple syrup

1 Tablespoon Coconut oil

1/4 teaspoon Chaga extract

¼ teaspoon Vanilla

1 Tablespoon Cacao paste

1 pinch of Himalayan salt

12 ounce container of ice (not heaping)

VEGAN

3 Tablespoons of cold Chaga tea

1 Tablespoon Coconut butter

1 Tablespoon Cacao powder

2 Tablespoons Maple syrup

1 Tablespoon Coconut oil

1/4 teaspoon Chaga extract

¼ teaspoon Vanilla

1 Tablespoon Cacao paste

1 pinch of Himalayan salt

3 Tablespoons Lucuma

½ teaspoon Sunflower or non-gmo Soy Lecithin

2 Tablespoons Brown Rice Protein powder

12 ounce container of ice (not heaping)

METHOD

Use a Vitamix blender.

Blend all ingredients except for Cacao nibs and ice.

Then blend in 12 ounces of ice. Top with Cacao nibs

WHEY

Whey is a low-temperature processed concentrated liquid, created from what remains after milk is turned into cheese. The best quality Whey, with the highest nutrition, will be from pasture-raised and grass-fed cows, and will be low-temperature dried. Whey protein is packed with amino acids for muscle nourishment, and for boosting energy. It is also high in calcium and phosphorus for bones, magnesium for nerves, and potassium for heart health.

In addition to its incredible food value and nutrient content, the role Whey plays in our Iced Alchemy is that it provides a rich, creamy base for flavour and texture (similar to an ice-cream). Colostrum can be substituted, if desired, or in the case of a vegan version, Brown Rice Protein powder. Each of these substitutes offers its own spectrum of nutrition.

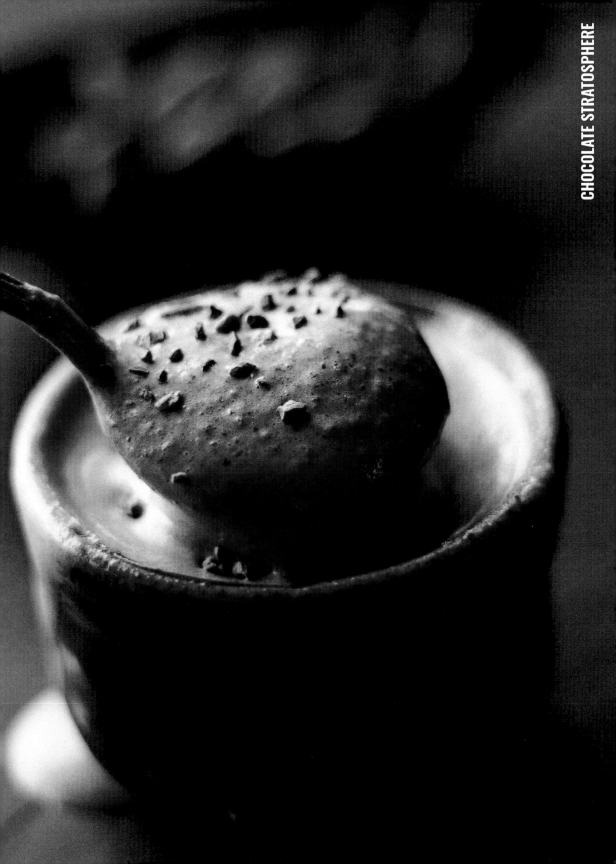

EARTH KISS

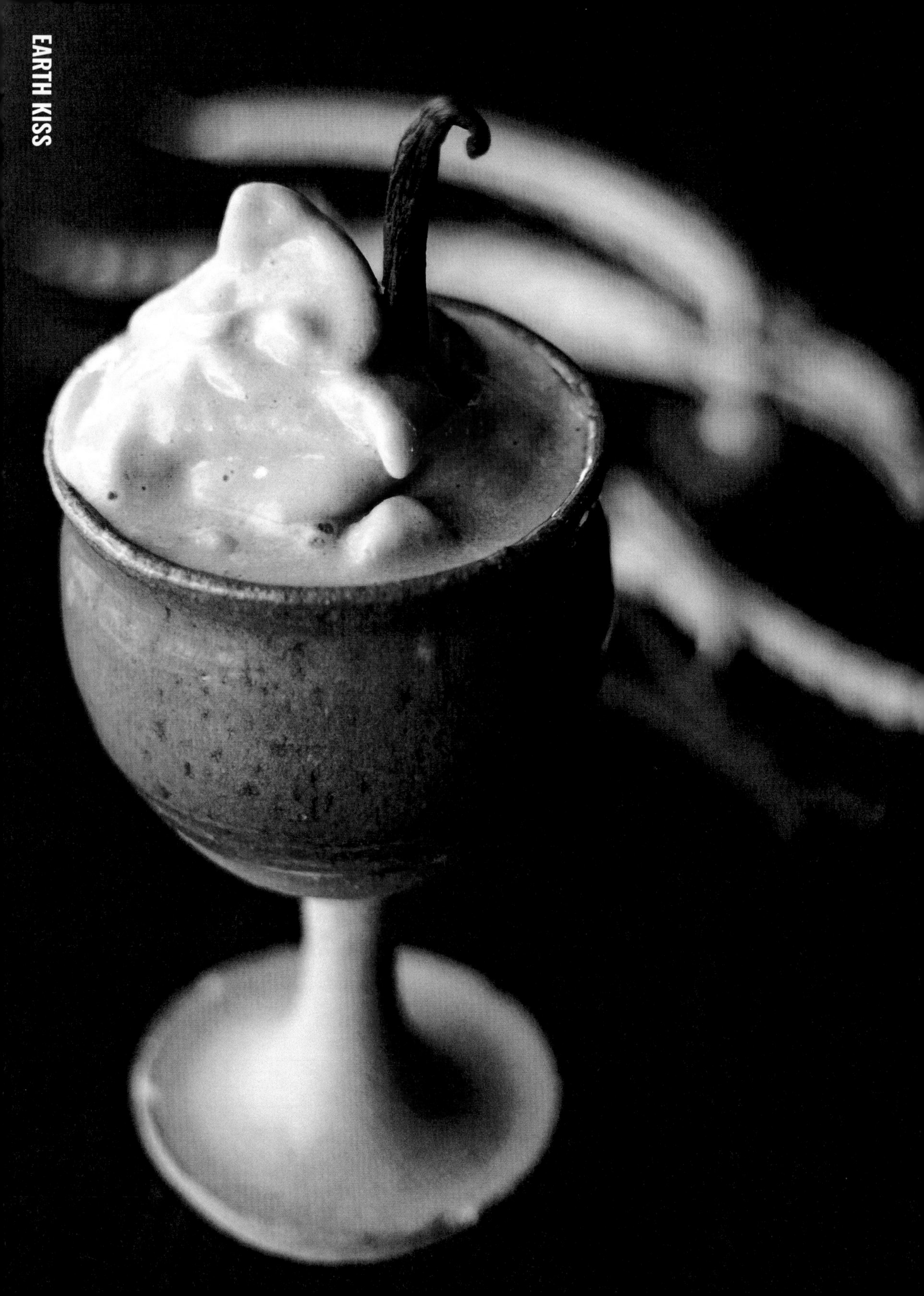

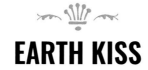

EARTH KISS

A tantalizing taste of golden malt flavors swirled with caramel earth tones.

INGREDIENTS

3 Tablespoons of cold Chaga tea

1 Tablespoon of Coconut butter

1 Tablespoon Maca powder

1 Tablespoon Mesquite powder

1 Tablespoon Lucuma powder

3 Tablespoons Whey

2 Tablespoons Maple syrup

¼ teaspoon Vanilla

1 pinch of Himalayan salt

12 ounce container of ice (not heaping)

VEGAN

3 Tablespoons of cold Chaga tea

1 Tablespoon Coconut butter

1 Tablespoon Maca powder

2 Tablespoon Mesquite powder

1 Tablespoon Lucuma powder

2 Tablespoon Maple syrup

¼ teaspoon Vanilla

1 pinch of Himalayan salt

½ teaspoon Sunflower or non-gmo Soy Lecithin

2 Tablespoons Brown Rice Protein powder

12 ounce container of ice (not heaping)

METHOD

Use a Vitamix blender.

Blend all ingredients except ice and then add in the ice and blend until smooth.

Serve with maple sugar topping or other garnish.

LUCUMA *Pouteria lucuma*

Pronounced loo-koo-ma. Lucuma is a delicious fruit that is native to the Andean valleys in South America. In ancestral times it was viewed as a symbol of fertility and creation, and was known as the 'Gold of the Incas'. Lucuma has a caramel, butterscotch, maple-like flavour that adds sweetness without a blood sugar spike. It has a soft taste and gentle aroma that enhances most Elixirs without overpowering in any way. Lucuma is high in beta-carotene for eyes and skin, fibre for regularity, and B3 for energy production.

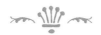

BERRY SUNRISE

A sun loving flight of berries.

INGREDIENTS

3 Tablespoons of cold Reishi or other tea

1 Tablespoon Coconut butter

3 Tablespoons Whey

1 Tablespoon Lucuma

2 Tablespoons Blueberry powder

1 Tablespoon Maqui or Acai powder

½ teaspoon Camu Camu

1 Tablespoon Baobab powder

2 drops Lemon oil

2 Tablespoons Honey

1 Tablespoon Cacao paste (optional)

¼ teaspoon Vanilla

1 pinch of Himalayan salt

12 ounce container of ice (not heaping)

VEGAN

3 Tablespoons of cold Reishi tea

1 Tablespoon Coconut butter

2 Tablespoons Lucuma

2 Tablespoons Blueberry powder

1 Tablespoon Maqui or Acai powder

½ teaspoon Camu Camu

1 Tablespoon Baobab powder

2 drops Lemon oil

2 Tablespoons Cane or Palm sugar

1 Tablespoon Cacao paste (optional)

¼ teaspoon Vanilla

1 pinch of Himalayan salt

½ teaspoon Sunflower or non-GMO Soy Lecithin

2 Tablespoons Brown Rice Protein powder

12 ounce container of ice (not heaping)

METHOD

Use a Vitamix blender.

Blend all ingredients except ice and then add in the ice and blend until smooth.

Serve in cup or bowl of choice with Cacao nibs, Bee pollen, or freeze dried fruit.

BAOBAB FRUIT POWDER *Adansonia spp*

The Baobab tree is considered the African 'Tree of Life'. It takes many years to fruit; most of the harvest comes from trees that have been standing for at least one hundred years. The fruit ripens and then completely dries on the branch before it is harvested, making it one of the only truly tree-ripened and sun-dried fruits in the world. Notable nutrients include potassium, iron, calcium, magnesium, phosphorus, and vitamin C. This fruit is also 50% fibre, soluble and insoluble, making it a great prebiotic—meaning a food which feeds your probiotics.

Baobab in the context of an Iced Alchemy, plays a role in offering a fruity, almost lemon-like flavour, and, of course, delivers its unique spectrum of nutrition. It also has the properties required to bring together and emulsify the liquid and fats in these creations, ensuring a creamy and smooth texture.

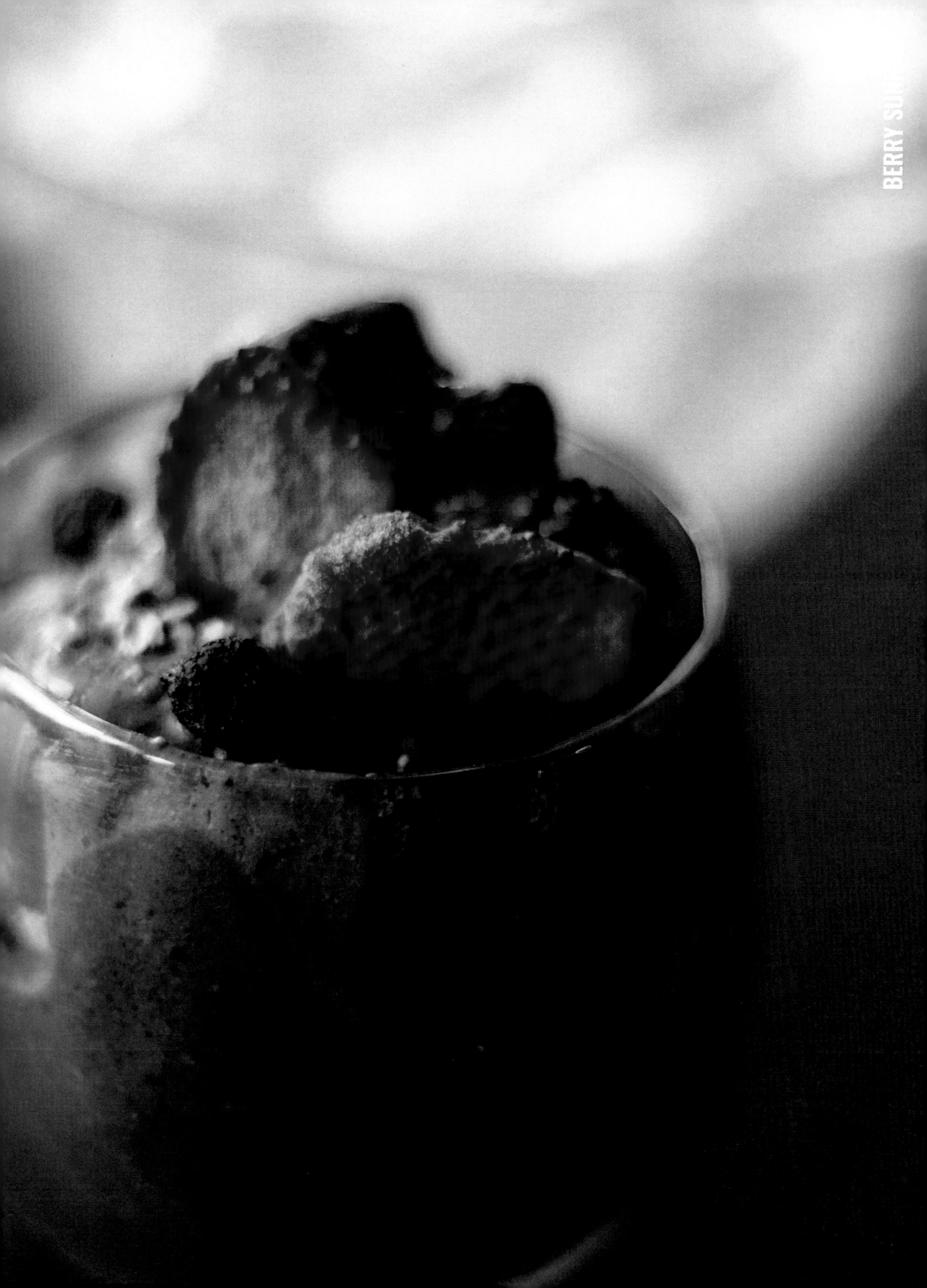

MYSTIC MOUNTAINTOP

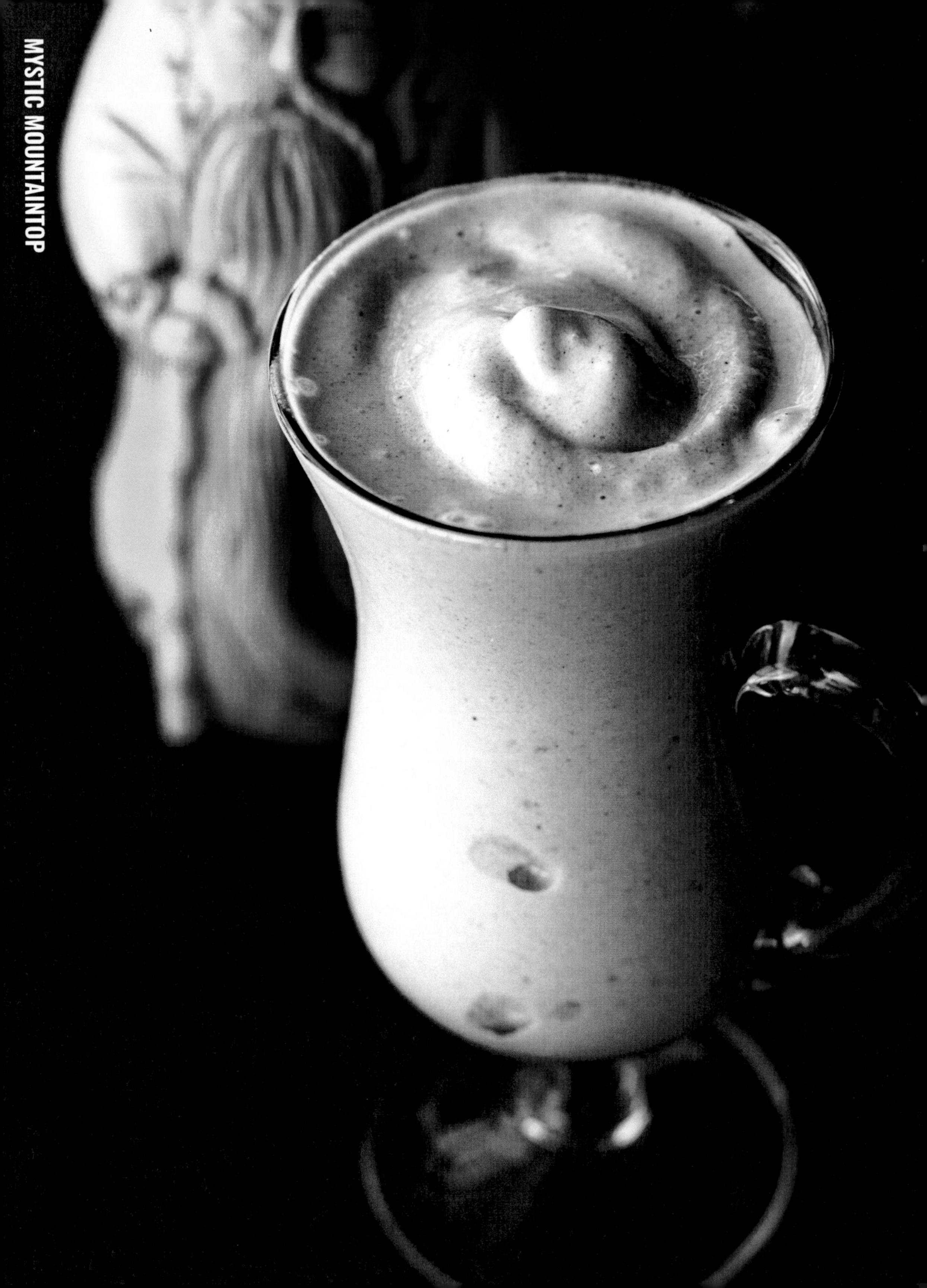

MYSTIC MOUNTAINTOP

A creamy alchemy with cheese-cake notes and a silver lining.

INGREDIENTS

3 Tablespoons of cold Chaga tea

1 Tablespoon Coconut butter

1 Tablespoon Coconut oil

4 Tablespoons Whey

2 Tablespoons Colostrum

1½ teaspoon Chai spice (optional)

1 Tablespoon Baobab powder

¼ cup toasted coconut flakes (optional)

2 Tablespoons Lucuma

2 teaspoons Colloidal Silver

2 Tablespoons Honey

¼ teaspoon Vanilla

1 pinch of Himalayan salt

12 ounce container of ice (not heaping)

METHOD

Use a Vitamix blender.

Blend all ingredients except for Cacao nibs and ice. When smooth, add ice and blend further.

Serve with Cacao nibs, or topping of choice

UPGRADE

Ginseng extract for extra energy

COLOSTRUM

Colostrum is known as the first milk or 'Immune Milk' produced by all mammal-mothers within the first few hours after birth. Considered regenerative, adaptogenic, and immuno-modulating Colostrum is a versatile, functional, whole food with many benefits and is easy to take and enjoy. This superfood is a complete protein, with a higher protein and fat content than regular milk, as well as fat-soluble vitamins, minerals, probiotics, growth-factors, and immunoglobulins. Before the development of antibiotics, colostrum was the main source for immunoglobulins used to fight bacteria. Colostrum contains 97 immune factors and 87 growth factors. It is known to support digestive health, help balance the intestinal system, and assist in repairing the nervous system. For best quality use only ethically sourced Colostrum from bovines, low temperature dried, and tested to be free of chemicals.

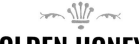

GOLDEN HONEYPOT

A subtly sweet honey taste and whole hive buzz.

INGREDIENTS

3 Tablespoons of cold Chaga tea

1 Tablespoon coconut butter

1 Tablespoon Coconut oil

3 Tablespoons Whey

2 Tablespoons Lucuma

2 Tablespoons Honey

¼ teaspoon Vanilla

40 drops Propolis tincture

1 Tablespoon Baobab

1 teaspoon Bee pollen

1 pinch Himalayan salt

12 ounce container of ice (not heaping)

VEGAN

3 Tablespoons of cold Chaga tea

1 Tablespoon Coconut butter

1 Tablespoon Coconut oil

3 Tablespoons Lucuma

2 Tablespoons Honey

¼ teaspoon Vanilla

40 drops Propolis tincture

1 Tablespoon Baobab

1 teaspoon Bee pollen

1 pinch Himalayan salt

2 Tablespoons Brown Rice Protein powder

12 ounce container of ice (not heaping)

METHOD

Use a Vitamix blender.

Blend all ingredients except Cacao nibs and/or Bee pollen. Once smooth, blend in ice. Serve in the cup of choice with cacao nibs and/or Bee pollen.

FOODS OF THE HIVE

Humans ought to be incredibly grateful to bees for all they provide. These wonderful little creatures make possible a large portion of our food chain through pollination of food crops, and they produce exquisitely tasting, nutrient dense and healing foods themselves—Honey, Bee Pollen, Propolis, and Royal Jelly. All the foods of the hive are full of nutrition and include a spectrum of vitamins and minerals. Bee foods are packed with Vitamin B, to help support the nervous system, and magnesium for muscles and heart health.

BEE POLLEN

Nature's fountain of youth, Bee pollen is often referred to as 'Ambrosia', a revered substance that bestows longevity. Bee pollen is a combination of the pollen gathered by bees from flowers as well as honey, and bee secretions. It's brought back to the hive as a primary food source for the young, nurse, and worker bees. Long consumed by humans, this longevity food is considered an energy and nutritive tonic in Chinese medicine. It has also been shown to be one of Nature's most complete and nourishing foods, containing nearly all nutrients required by humans, providing over 95 essential elements for the body. It is a high source of protein for cell building, and high in iron for energy and blood strengthening. Bee pollen is also rich in enzymes to aid in digestion and helps absorb nutrients.

Start small with Bee pollen, to make sure you have no sensitivities or allergies to it; some do. If new to Bee pollen try 1/8 teaspoon and gradually increase to 1-2 teaspoons.

Bee pollen is contraindicated in hypertension and diabetes, and should be crushed thoroughly to ensure benefit.

PROPOLIS

Propolis, known as 'bee glue' or the 'defense of the city', is a resinous substance bees use to fill crevices in the hive. It is considered the external immune system of the hive. Propolis is made by the bees from a mixture of beeswax, bee saliva, and exudate of tree buds, sap flows, and other botanical sources. Though you can find Propolis as a resin and chew it like a gum, it is best used in tincture form. The pure, raw resin is placed in a high-percentage alcohol to extract all the nutrients and benefits. It is easy to use. Propolis has been used for thousands of years in traditional medicine for a variety of conditions including as an alternative to antibiotics to fight infection and help the healing process. This superfood contains nearly all the nutrients required by the body.

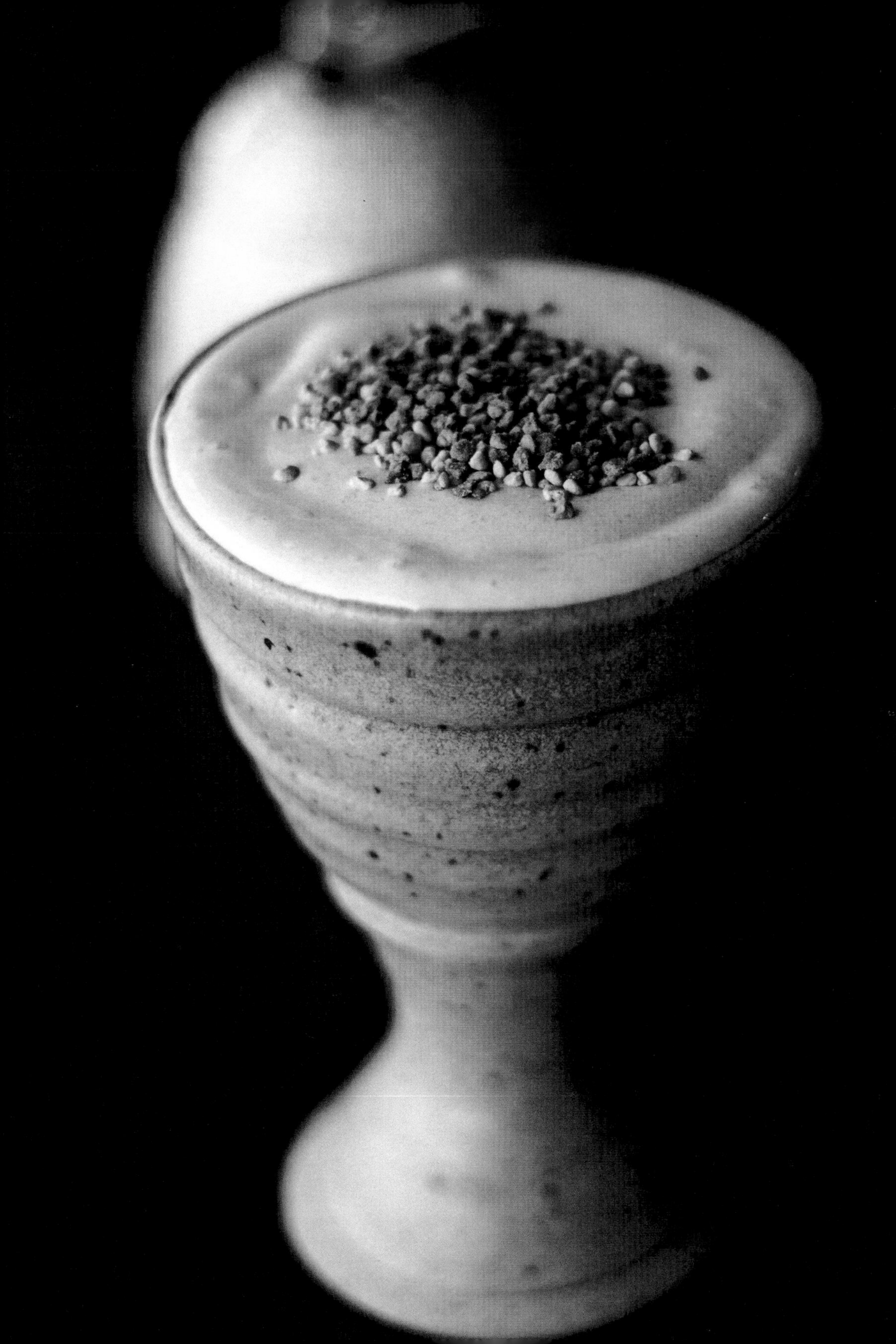

THE LIGHT CELLAR

The Light Cellar is a place where you can find, and learn how to craft, your own food and medicine.

We are an independent and inspired business offering the largest range of superfoods in Canada.

When you visit, you will receive care, guidance, and expertise. You will be able to select from the highest quality superfoods, superherbs, medicinal mushrooms, friendly ferments, chocolate making ingredients, and more. You can also enjoy a hot or cold Elixir.

We envision a world that honours the sacredness of all life and source only the best, highest quality ingredients which have been wild-crafted or grown at or above organic standards. We offer ongoing classes, events, and workshops to support you in your journey to sustainably and deliciously nourish your being.

THE STORY OF TLC

The Light Cellar began in the basement of Laura's parents' house—she and I (Malcolm) lived there for a short time—after post-secondary schooling and post-world-travels—while we figured out our next direction in life. We were young and motivated to help change the world, while improving our own lives.

At that time, both Laura and I had been vegetarians for more than a decade, and I'd been immersed in the world of raw veganism. My passion for health, food, and nutrition was extreme. It directed my everyday decision making, and soon took me and my new family South to work at a raw-vegan retreat centre in Arizona.

A constant striving to learn, and try new things, led to an expanded repertoire in the kitchen.

I was compelled to find a diet that reflected my own philosophical approach to life, while meeting my real physical nutritional needs. I evolved and moved away from vegetarianism.

My deep dive into the world of plant-based foods led me to superfoods, medicinal mushrooms, and eventually to herbal traditions from around the world. Ultimately, that led to discovering Elixirs and their further development. It was my experience with the significant personal impact and changes from superfoods that inspired me to share with others. I started by teaching workshops out of our basement; in those early days, a group of sometimes six or less was a success.

I began ordering bulk amounts of my favourite superfoods to the house because supply and availability in Calgary was scarce. I knew what I wanted in terms of selection and quality; I just couldn't find it. From living

in the States, I had names of suppliers, and so I began ordering—first for my own use. I soon added a couple extra pounds to my orders for friends, and for those taking classes.

We never planned or envisioned opening a store, but it evolved naturally. Initially, when Laura and I got our own home, we set up the basement to house her colonic practice, and for me to host classes, and to produce small, saleable quantities from bulk orders. We joked about being a "feed 'em and clean 'em" operation. In addition, we opened our home for anyone to come by on a Sunday to pick up some items, and chat.

Word of mouth has always been our best strategy for growing our business, yet at this time it was hindered because of the circumstances. People would say that they loved what we offered, and would tell their friends about us, jokingly referring to us as their 'dealer'. The instructions given to their friends to go 'around the back of this dude's house to his basement to get the goods' wasn't always met with enthusiasm or eagerness.

So, after a year and a half, back in 2007, we made the leap and rented a very small commercial space on Bowness Road in Northwest Calgary, a location in which we have grown and expanded.

Since the beginning, while all this was unfolding, equally part of my joy and my offering was making chocolate. Born out of my love for playing in the kitchen, experimenting with recipes, and always trying to upgrade the familiar to something more healthy and extraordinary, I had developed a reputation for my tasty and healthy superfood-filled chocolate cups. To this day, they are still produced by the Light Cellar.

What was originally chocolate-making extended to fermentation—sauerkraut. The next stop was Elixirs.

In the early days of Elixir Crafting, we featured a weekly special Elixir. Created on a whim, influenced by season and whatever ingredients we had on hand, our customers would order one of these warm elixirs when they stopped in for weekly supplies. We'd blend the Elixirs in the back while our customers shopped.

It was during renovations, a few years in, that we created an Elixir bar with a full menu of offerings that included warm and cold Elixirs. It was one of North America's first Elixir bars. The recipes in this book are a compilation of our best. We have continually refined and upgraded the recipes, improving them, not only in taste and experience, but also in efficiency and cost. We have come a long way, and are very pleased to offer you this book so you can bring Elixirs into your life.

EPILOGUE

Your body, and its inherent wisdom, holds the secret to achieving vibrant health.

It's important to me that my offerings are practical, attainable, and sustainable.

It is my pleasure to help you connect to your food more deeply so that you can benefit from the sacred goodness of eating, creating, and sharing.

An invitation to follow me and the Light Cellar on Instagram and Facebook remains open. I am **@themalchemist**. You can use and follow the hashtag #elixirlife — I'd be stoked to see your creations.

I'd love it if you visit the Light Cellar YouTube channel to view the "Easy Upgrade" videos created to help empower and inspire you in the kitchen. There, along with special guests and experts, you will find simple recipes and concepts to add to your repertoire.

For any ingredients you need, visit us in-store. Stay awhile and enjoy an Elixir, check out the books we carry, and take your time browsing. Not in town? Can't make it to the store? Email or give us a call.

And, definitely come join me in a class. I'll walk you through the basics of developing and trusting your own wisdom and skills in the area of food and nutrition.

Enjoy the Elixir Life
Craft the Life of Your Dreams

Malcolm Saunders

CLASSES AND EVENTS AT THE LIGHT CELLAR

Empowering educational experiences to enlighten your culinary abilities, and expand your perspectives about food and nutrition

The Light Cellar Learning Kitchen is a friendly place to begin or continue your journey of health. Our classes are designed to meet you where you're at, and help you to easily upgrade your understanding and approach to food and nutrition.

By attending classes at the Light Cellar you will gain knowledge, new skills, and perhaps most importantly, the confidence to know how to provide more deeply nourishing food for yourself and your family.

Check out our current list of classes. Registration is online. You will find a diversity of topics from expert instructors.

"My quest has been to learn about various foods that have high nutritional value or about specific techniques and TLC has been the ideal, hands-on learning classroom for me." - Lindsay P.

"My main reason for coming to the classes is to stretch out from what I already do and to incorporate more nutrition into our (family's) diet. I now have the confidence to make sauerkraut, and will be incorporating more super greens in chocolates, in ice cream... I really enjoyed the many classes and talks that I have been to." - Janice S.

"I like the variety of topics presented and the range from the practical to the philosophical. I like the mix of demo, hands-on and discussion in the way classes are presented.

This shows me I don't need to be perfect or get it right all at once. It is a journey and I can traverse in stages. Very useful information on nutritive qualities and health functions of specific superfoods and herbs and ways to incorporate them into my life with recipes and cooking suggestions. This has helped me in deciding what foods/herbs to add to my diet at this time to support certain health concerns." - Donna B.

"I love how these classes take ingredients that border the arcane (understood by few; mysterious or secret) and translate them into approachable, normal, and easy." - Janis I.

"I love the classes and the atmosphere" - Theresa C.

"I had an extraordinary time and feel so grateful for this information and exposure! I am SO ready to include this 'fermentation' in my family's foods... and on this path to wellness and balance it feels essential... So thank you... I am already scheming for what other classes I can participate in...

Oh, and of course, the 'hands on' takes absorbing the info to another level and I really dug that.

You Light Cellar people are super lovely! Right on for all you put out there.

Thank you, thank you!" - Lora D.

"You expanded my repertoire of food and showed me the world of superfoods. I have so enjoyed your classes, they are like an oasis" - Alison L.

"The experiential learning has enabled me to leave a class and integrate the learning into my life right away. I have received an expanded awareness of the properties, history and folklore that surround the products being presented." - Matt M.

I BELIEVE

I believe food is sacred, healing, and beautiful. I use it to uplift the experience of each day.

I believe eating food is one of the most intimate relationships we have with the natural word.

I believe in keeping food as natural as possible because what we eat literally becomes our body, and I've experienced how different foods, good and bad, can affect mind and emotions.

I believe that food which is good for my body is also good for the Earth.

I believe my food choices have the power to help make the world a better place.

THE PATH

Health, through nutrition, is a personal journey; it's about nourishing yourself and those you love.

It's about listening to your body, exploring what works, and feeling what doesn't.

I've personally experimented with many dietary paths, trying on, and testing what might work.

Today, I follow my gut more than I follow nutrition trends.

I feel really positive about my health and the relationship I have to food.

IT WASN'T ALWAYS THIS WAY

When I first began this journey I knew nothing.

Sixteen years old; could make grilled cheese, heat microwave pizza, and toast Pop Tarts.

STILL IN MY TEENS

I knew I could do better, and that I could feel good from the food I ate.

I became interested in recreating my relationship to food.

I just didn't know how to do it, or where to start.

TODAY

In addition to being a husband and dad, I am the founder, owner, and creative visionary of the Light Cellar, considered to be one of the premier superfood stores in North America.

My journey, and all that I have learned along the route, is what I share.

What can be enjoyed most at the Light Cellar is the sense of community, connection, non-judgement, and the atmosphere of comfort so that anyone can learn and grow with new knowledge, friends, and foods.

ONE OF MY PASSIONS IS TEACHING

My workshops and seminars have helped thousands recreate their relationship with food.

I am continuing this work by writing books, creating e-courses, getting on stage, and filming 'how-to' videos.

My passion is to provide others with insight into a variety of topics, from the practical to the philosophical.

Educating and inspiring individuals to gain confidence in their own health journey, learn new life-skills, and feel empowered, is intensely rewarding.

WHY I DO WHAT I DO

To help others get a little further, more easily, and without all the U-turns, circles, and dead-ends I experienced.

To simplify food science and nutritional information for others.

To guide a return to basics, to whole nutrient-dense foods, prepared healthily.

To honour my own relationship with the planet.

ABOUT THE AUTHOR:

Malcolm Saunders' mission is to deeply connect people to their food. He has worked in the field of food and nutrition for close to twenty years, and is the Owner and Creative Visionary of the Light Cellar. Malcolm is a public speaker and an intuitive chef who specializes in sharing the alchemy of superfoods and superherbs. Through his videos, workshops, and seminars he has helped thousands of individuals recreate their relationship to food. He has an expertise and passion for creating and teaching others how to make energizing and healing foods, including chocolate, Elixirs, and ferments.

Malcolm's desire is to inspire others to live and eat from a space that honours the sacredness of all Life, illuminating the powerful influence our food choices have on us, other beings, and the planet. A passionate advocate for intuitive eating, he has created events, and shared the stage with world-renowned speakers including David Wolfe, Daniel Vitalis, Sandor Katz, Nadine Artemis, and Dr. Terry Willard. You can find his work at malcolmsaunders.com

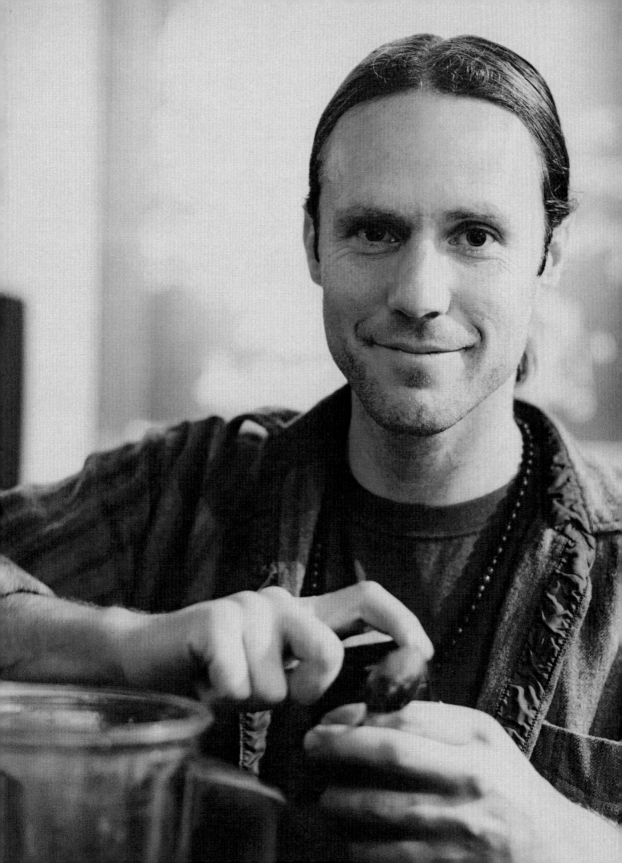